NURSING
REVISION NOTES

SURGICAL
NURSING

NURSING
REVISION NOTES

SURGICAL
NURSING

by
M. J. Jenkins SRN; DN(London); RCNT; RNT; Cert.Ed.; M.Ed.
and
L. Moran SRN; DN(London); RCNT; RNT; Cert.Ed.; B.Ed.

CELTIC
REVISION AIDS

Celtic Revision Aids
30-32 Gray's Inn Road
London WC1X 8JL

© C.E.S.

First published 1982
Reprinted 1983 (twice)

ISBN 0 86305 122 7

Printed and bound in Great Britain by
Collins, Glasgow

GENERAL EDITOR'S FOREWORD

The nursing revision series is designed for all nurses in training. The notes are suitable for pre-modular study, post-modular revision and examination revision, and will also be of value to learners undertaking ongoing assessment. While being comprehensive in the major areas of both patient condition and nursing care, they are intended to complement, not replace, existing text books. Each book provides information on basic anatomy and physiology, aspects of investigations and nursing care and practice questions and answers are included at the end of each section. The authors have used their experience in nurse education to select important areas of nursing care for inclusion and I am sure that all nurse learners will find the books of continuing value throughout their training.

P. J. Morland
Lecturer
Department of Education
University College Cardiff

AUTHORS' FOREWORD

These notes are intended for nurse learners taking the module of surgical experience, and for learners revising for hospital and state final examinations.

The aim of this revision guide is to help nurse learners to test their knowledge and understanding of:

a Regional and applied anatomy and physiology
b Investigation and treatment of patients who may undergo surgery
c Reasons for specific management.

The authors have been selective in content, only common problems needing surgical intervention have been included, this is dictated by the length and scope of the text.

Each section sets out common problems experienced by individuals suffering from particular disease processes. We have set out normal and abnormal body functions as a basis for understanding. The important clinical features of disease processes are set out together with the specific investigations necessary to establish diagnosis and management.

The sections are concluded with a range of tests and situations designed to test knowledge, comprehension and application. Answers are provided to check against. Advice for preparation for examinations and examination techniques are included at the end of the book.

CONTENTS

INTRODUCTION

The surgical situation — some nursing considerations

Many people are admitted to hospital for operations. The 'operation' is often seen as a traumatic event by the patient and his family and at the time often clouds all other events. However the nurse should remember that for the majority of patients, the period spent in hospital before and after the operation, not only constitutes a very short period in the patient's life but constitutes a short period in the span of that particular illness. With this in mind, it is inappropriate to think of the patient and his condition in isolation, it becomes essential to think of them both in terms of the patient as an individual, and as a member of a family and as a member of society.

Operations may be of a minor or of a major nature. The person undergoing the operation **may have had time to prepare** for their admission to hospital, may have had weeks or even months to arrange their lives and families to 'fit in' with his or her hospitalization, alternatively, the patient may have been admitted to hospital in **an emergency situation** with no, or very little, time to prepare.

Again, the patient may have the capacity **to understand fully** what his hospitalization will involve, **be fully aware** of the nature of the condition which warrants surgery, have the personality to question **anything** he does not understand and possess the ability and/or willingness **to discuss and accept** his progress or otherwise with those looking after him and with his relatives. On the other hand, the person may **be unable or unwilling to understand or do** any of these things.

For a nurse to be effective it is necessary for her to care for each patient as an **individual,** who has specific needs and reactions to a particular condition. She must of course be aware of the diagnosis and condition of the person but she must consider carefully its **particular** effect. In other words, how does the patient's condition (illness) affect him, his daily living activities, his usual pattern of life, his level of independence.

Each individual copes with their daily living activities in their own way. When we are not ill we cope with these activities with minimum dependence on others, indeed when we are well we are probably not even aware of our dependence on, or independence of, others. So, when we become ill we do not think of our illness in the medical sense, we think of it in terms of how it affects our particular lifestyle or daily living

1

activities. Your patient is not, therefore, so much interested in the fact that he has a duodenal ulcer with pyloric stenosis (other than knowing that the doctors know what is wrong with him), but rather in the fact that he cannot enjoy his meals anymore without feeling pain and discomfort, he suffers from nausea and vomiting, and his general feeling of being unwell makes him irritable with his family and unable to concentrate on his work. Similarly, he is not so much interested in the technicalities of the surgical procedure that he is to undergo, but how the outcome of the operation will affect him.

The illness is thought of in terms of his ability or inability to cope with the normal life pattern, in terms of the help needed to carry out specific functions. The hospitalization is also defined in terms of what he will be able or be allowed to do for himself and what he will be dependent on others for. Too often in the past the nurse has considered her nursing care in terms of how much she can do for the patient rather than how much the patient could do for himself if he had the appropriate nursing help. We do the patient a disservice when even out of kindness we 'do everything for him'. Not only do we take away his independence when he is in hospital, we take away the opportunity for him to achieve previously determined goals from day to day and we also limit the use of the post-operative period for an individually based rehabilitation programme.

The nurse is equipped with a basic knowledge of principles of care and with nursing skills when she is allocated to the surgical ward for experience. When she considers the patients with their various conditions who may be on a general surgical ward at any given time, she is able to see that the **basic principles of surgical nursing apply to them all.** To explain . . . they all need preparation for surgery, they all need assistance of some sort in the post-operative period, they all need to be carefully observed and so on . . . what the nurse must do **is discriminate between the specific needs of each** of the patients in her care.

1 GENERAL PRINCIPLES OF PRE- AND POST-OPERATIVE NURSING CARE

The general principles of pre- and post-operative nursing care are included at the outset so that they can be established and used as a source of reference. Specific nursing care will be referred to in the text.

Before applying the basic principles of care to any particular patient, the nurse should first consider the events which have led to the patient being considered for operation.

Type of admission

Planned
a From a waiting list.

b From another ward or hospital where specific treatment has commenced

Emergency
a From home or work, via the GP or emergency services (sudden event).

b Via the GP or consultant domiciliary visit following a period of illness at home.

c Via Outpatient clinic which the patient has been attending.

d Transfer from another ward or hospital where the patient is being treated for the same or a different condition.

Reason for admission
a The person has an acute condition which can only be best relieved by surgery.

b Medical treatment has failed or is not controlling the disease process.

c The individual's psychological well-being is at stake.

Type of operation
a **Major** — one stage

b **Multistage** — this may be necessary because:
   i the general condition of the patient is too poor to cope with more extensive surgery at one time.
   ii An organ or cavity needs to be rested or drained as a preliminary to full operation.

c **Minor**

The nurse in the surgical ward is often confused by the variations in treatment and care of surgical patients that are ordered by different surgeons. However, a knowledge of basic principles will help her understand that even though methods may differ from surgeon to surgeon, the basic principles of care still apply.

Pre-operation

The main aim of pre-operative preparation is to render the patient as fit as possible for operation. The medical/nursing team may have days or weeks in which to do this, or may have only an hour or so. During this time, the patient's fitness to undergo anaesthesia and withstand any operation will be assessed. It should be possible to discover any other disturbances in the patient's general condition or physical state which may complicate the operation. If found, appropriate corrective treatment may be ordered.

Initial examination

All patients admitted to the surgical ward will have a careful history taken and have a full physical examination.

Depending on the diagnosis, date/time of operation and general condition of the patient, the doctor will then order that certain investigations be carried out. Some of these will be routine investigations carried out on all patients, and others will be special investigations appropriate to the patient's condition and planned operation.

The nurse should be familiar with what is routine, and have a basic understanding of the specific investigations that may be required.

Particular note is made of any drugs which the patient has been taking and a decision is made as to whether these drugs should be continued, whether a different drug regime be prescribed, or whether all drugs will be stopped. It may be appropriate during or following the initial examination to ask the patient to sign the relevant consent-for-operation form. This is the doctor's responsibility, the nurse should however be aware of the different consent forms used.

Psychological factors

Getting to know her patient and giving him every opportunity to discuss any particular fears and anxieties, is an important part of the nurse's function. Being able to deal with some of a patient's problems and knowing when to refer others to people better able to help, is also important. Explanation of procedures, passing on relevant information to patients and their relatives and explaining what to expect on the day of operation and following operation, have been proven to help the patient recover more quickly from the operation.

Nutrition

The patient should be rendered in as good a nutritional state as possible. A high protein, high calorie, easily digestible diet with vitamin supplements may be necessary. If the patient is unable to eat and time allows, intravenous feeding may even be ordered to improve the patient's nutritional state before surgery.

Fluid and electrolyte imbalance should be corrected, again, if necessary by intravenous replacement.

Blood loss may be replaced by blood transfusion.

Anaemia should be corrected by an oral regime if time allows or blood transfusion if not.

Withholding oral food and fluid for approximately 6 hours is sufficient for most people undergoing anaesthesia. In an emergency, if the patient has eaten in the previous 4 hours, the stomach may need to be washed out to lessen the risk of vomiting.

Specifically, with some gastro-intestinal surgery, the surgeon may wish the gut to be clear, in these instances only a fluid diet is allowed for some days prior to operation — this usually combines with a specific bowel preparation regime.

Bowel action

Generally, if the patient has had no bowel action on the day preceding surgery, suppositories may need to be used to encourage an action.

An evacuant enema may sometimes be necessary, although routine use of these has ceased. For specific operations on the gastro-intestinal tract, the bowel will need to be specifically prepared. This preparation might be a combination of oral bowel antiseptics taken for up to 5 days pre-operatively; mechanical preparation i.e. an enema followed by rectal washout once or twice daily for 2-4 days and a fluid diet for the same period as the mechanical bowel preparation.

Urine test

All patients undergoing surgery must have their urine routinely tested. It may be necessary to send specimens to the laboratory for analysis, culture and sensitivity.

Breathing and general exercises

Any respiratory infections are treated with antibiotics. If the patient has a productive cough, a specimen of sputum will be sent for laboratory examination. The patient is strongly advised to give up smoking. The physiotherapist is informed of the pending surgery and teaches the patient how to breath correctly, how to expectorate effectively and any special exercises appropriate to the particular operation which the patient will have to perform in the post-operative period. The patient is kept as fully mobile as possible until the time of operation, and informed at this stage of the importance of early mobilization after operation.

Hygiene and preparation of skin

General cleanliness of the skin is vital. This does not pose too much of a problem if the patient is admitted some days prior to surgery, but in the emergency situation, immediate resuscitative measures and the condition of the patient will need to be taken into consideration.

Usually, the patient is shaved and has a general bath or bed bath on the day before the operation. Particular attention should be paid to the nails and umbilicus. The area of skin to be shaved varies with each operation but each surgeon will issue his own instructions.

The day of operation, as part of the immediate pre-operative care, the patient will be bathed again, and instructed to remove nail varnish, not to use make-up, perfume or talcum powder etc.

The operation site is checked again by the nurse and the patient is then dressed in an operation gown and cap.

Immediate pre-operative check

Most hospitals have devised a check list which can be used for this. These forms usually facilitate checking the following:

Site of operation properly prepared.
Specific preparations have been carried out.
Whether urine has been passed and when.
Last recorded temperature.
Prosthesis have been removed.
Premedication has been given and time administered.
Identification of patient.
Appropriate notes, X-rays, pathology reports are available.
Consent form completed.

Post-operation

Post-operative care begins whilst the patient is still undergoing operation. The bed area is prepared with any additional features the nurse considers will be required when the patient returns from theatre. She will need to know what operation has been planned and is being performed and the expected condition of the patient.

On arrival at the recovery area of theatre, the nurse should identify herself, her ward and the patient she is to collect. Before leaving the recovery area, she should make sure she is in possession of all the necessary information regarding the operation, surgeon, condition of the patient during and following operation and any instructions regarding his care for the immediate post-operative period.

Before escorting the patient back to the ward, she should:

a check the emergency equipment on the theatre trolley.

b see that the patient's condition is satisfactory to take back to the ward.

c check that the patient is safely on the trolley.

d check that any infusions, drainage apparatus etc. are safe and in working order.

As soon as possible after arriving back on the ward, the nurse should pass on all relevant information to the nurse in charge.

Position of the patient

It is customary nowadays for patients to remain in the recovery area of theatre until they have regained consciousness, are responding to commands and their condition is regarded as stable.

The position in which to nurse the patient in the immediate period following return to the ward will depend, therefore, on:

a the level of consciousness.

b level and stability of vital signs.

c site and type of wound — there should be minimum tension and pressure.

d position and type of drainage — position such that maximum drainage is promoted and security and safety of drainage apparatus is ensured.

e whether patient is to be attached to any apparatus e.g. traction.

f any special instructions from medical staff.

Observations

It is very important that the patient's condition be assessed and recorded immediately he is transferred into his bed if it is to be used as a baseline from which subsequent recordings can be compared.

The following should be noted:

Temperature.

Pulse (rate, rythym, volume).

Respiration (rate, depth, character).

Blood pressure.

Level of consciousness and response of patient.

Colour and texture of skin.

Wound site, type of dressing (any evidence of blood loss).

Wound drainage site, type of apparatus (amount and description of drainage fluid).

The degree, site and type of pain, if present.

Intravenous regime.

Presence of any other tubes in situ e.g. nasogastric, catheters.

Amount and type of fluid draining (whether they are to be on free or intermittent drainage).

The frequency of which general and specific observations are to be recorded will be established as soon as the patient has been settled in bed. They will be monitored and changed in response to the progress, or otherwise, of the patient.

Pain relief

Post-operative analgesia is likely to be prescribed by the anaesthetist to cover at least the first 24-48 hours, after which dosage is usually reduced. It is usually prescribed for 4-6 hourly intervals to be given if necessary. The patient should not be allowed to experience any more than the minimum amount of pain, thus analgesia should be given regularly.

However, to be effective analgesia should be given in conjunction with nursing procedures and patient activity e.g. physiotherapy and mobilisation programme. Careful attention should also be given to the position of the patient, wounds and any drainage tubes, since tension or pressure on the wound and badly placed drainage apparatus can cause the patient undue discomfort. Observations of the patient are recorded before and after administration and the effect of the drug noted.

Nausea and vomiting

Any patient may experience nausea and vomiting following anaesthesia and even the most minor surgery. This can be very distressing. The nurse should remain with the patient if he is vomiting, providing a clean receiver, tissues, change of bedwear, and mouth care as necessary. Any vomitus should be measured and description recorded. If vomiting persists, an anti-emitic may be prescribed and in some instances nasogastric aspiration instituted.

Nutrition and fluids

Many patients will return from theatre and will have no restriction on oral intake of food and fluid once the immediate post-operative period is over. The nurse should check therefore:

a how soon the patient is allowed to eat and/or drink.

b the nature and volume of what is allowed (in some instances e.g. prostatectomy, it is necessary to encourage fluids as soon as the patient can tolerate them, in an attempt to encourage urinary drainage.

Following many operations on the gastro-intestinal tract, however, there is a restriction on oral intake. The patient returns from theatre with an intravenous infusion/transfusion and a nasogastric tube *in situ*. Following these operations, the gut undergoes a period of stasis and peristaltic action is diminished or lost for a period which may last up to 2-4 days. (Bowel sounds are absent — the patient does not pass flatus, there may be some gaseous distension). Secretions cannot pass through the gut and would accumulate causing possible nausea and vomiting and gastric dilatation. The stomach is therefore kept empty by means of the nasogastric drainage. The nurse should find out:

a whether aspirations should be performed at timed intervals.

b whether a drainage bag be attached to the nasogastric tube, thus allowing continuous drainage.

The intravenous infusion is necessary to:

a replace fluids lost during and following surgery (a record is kept of intravenous regime given during the operation and recovery period, and usually the anaesthetist issues instructions regarding the regime to cover the immediate period following return to ward).

b maintain fluid and electrolyte balance during the period of restricted intake. Usually the intravenous regime is prescribed by the doctor each day, in response to daily serum urea and electrolyte levels and estimation of previous days fluid balance.

During the period of restricted oral intake, nasal and oral care is performed as necessary. The patient may be allowed ice or sweets to suck.

Oral fluids are usually recommended between 24-72 hours when:

a bowel sounds have returned.

b gastric aspirations have decreased.

c flatus is being passed.

d abdomen is soft.

Oral fluids are then increased gradually, nasogastric tube removed. Fluids continue to be increased and infusion is discontinued when adequate oral fluids are being tolerated.

Urinary output

The nurse should take particular note of whether the patient has passed urine or not since the operation and record the information accordingly. If not, it is important to establish whether the patient has post-operative retention or suppression of urine.

The patient may experience a temporary inability to void:

a due to the effects of drugs or trauma in the bladder region, which cause depression of bladder sensitivity to distention.

b inability to relax because of discomfort, pain and anxiety.

Retention with overflow when small amounts of urine are voided frequently, results from distension of the bladder.

If the patient has not passed urine for 8-12 hours, the doctor should be informed. Bladder catheterisation may be considered to be necessary as a last resort.

Activity/early ambulation

In order to minimise the risk of chest infection and possible lung collapse, as soon as the patient has fully recovered from the anaesthetic, deep breathing exercises are encouraged. Correct positioning, support of wounds and adequate analgesia will help ensure that this is effective. A persistent cough — apart from tiring the patient, puts an undue strain on an abdominal wound which could lead to delayed wound healing.

Whilst in bed, frequent change of position and movement of limbs is carried out (passive physiotherapy) or encouraged (active physiotherapy) in order to minimise the risk of joint stiffness and vascular complications.

This general movement also helps prevent flatulence, abdominal distension and urinary retention.

Within 24-48 hours, if his condition is satisfactory, the patient is assisted out of bed and encouraged to walk about. The degree of mobilisation at this time varies with each patient and is increased in relation to the patient's general response and progress.

2 THE OESOPHAGUS

The objectives of chapters 2, 3, 4 and 5 are to state the following.
1   The regional and applied structure and function of the alimentary canal (excluding the mouth).
2   The diseases most commonly occurring in the alimentary canal and the ways in which they interfere with normal function.
3   The management of the individual undergoing investigation and treatment of conditions of the alimentary canal.

Fig. 1, overleaf, shows a diagrammatic representation of the position and shape of the abdominal organs. Please revise thoroughly with the aid of textbooks, models and your lecture notes. Learn to draw the diagrams and label them correctly.

The oesophagus

The oesophagus is a hollow fibro-muscular tube about 25 cm long. It is lined with epithelial tissue and extends from the cricopharyngeal sphincter through the posterior mediastinum and diaphragm to the cardiac sphincter of the stomach. Nerve supply is mediated via,
a   the vagus nerve (parasympathetic system).
b   Auerbach's plexus (these nerve elements are defective in the condition called **achalasia** or **cardio-spasm**).
The portal or systemic veins anastomose (or join) at the lower third of the oesophagus. Back pressure on these veins causes them to dilate, a condition named oesophageal varices. Oesophageal or gastric varices (varicose veins) may be caused by portal hypertension (raised pressure in the portal vein) caused by:
a   cirrhosis of the liver in 80% of cases.
b   congenital abnormality of the portal vein.
c   thrombosis of the portal vein.

Precipitating factors of bleeding varices

When there is increased pressure causing the dilated walls of the veins to burst.
When the veins are continually battered with regurgitated gastric juice.
When a food bolus causes trauma to the weakened vessels. A slow or massive haemorrhage can occur.

Fig 1

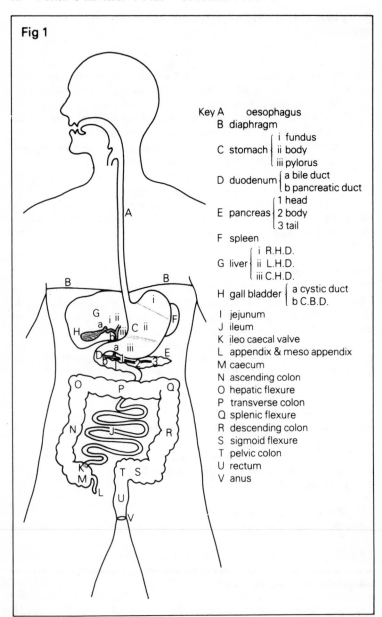

Key A   oesophagus
B diaphragm

C stomach { i fundus / ii body / iii pylorus

D duodenum { a bile duct / b pancreatic duct

E pancreas { 1 head / 2 body / 3 tail

F spleen

G liver { i R.H.D. / ii L.H.D. / iii C.H.D.

H gall bladder { a cystic duct / b C.B.D.

I jejunum
J ileum
K ileo caecal valve
L appendix & meso appendix
M caecum
N ascending colon
O hepatic flexure
P transverse colon
Q splenic flexure
R descending colon
S sigmoid flexure
T pelvic colon
U rectum
V anus

The physiology of swallowing occurs in two phases. (The tissue is specially adapted for this, see Fig 2).

1 the voluntary phase of swallowing
2 the involuntary stage of swallowing

1 The voluntary phase begins as food is pressed between the tongue and soft palate. It is flipped back into the pharynx and the soft palate moves back and upwards to block the naso pharynx. (Failure of this mechanism results in regurgitation of food through the nose, a distressing problem that occurs in myasthenia gravis — a condition of neuro muscular dysfunction). The epiglottis lifts over the glottis and the larynx blocking the airway, breathing is momentarily inhibited and food passes into oesophagus. (Failure of this mechanism results in inhalation of food mucus or saliva. This is a problem that may occur from damage to the brain involving the swallowing centre and in myasthenia gravis). The unconscious person is particularly vulnerable to inhale mucus and saliva, this

Fig 2

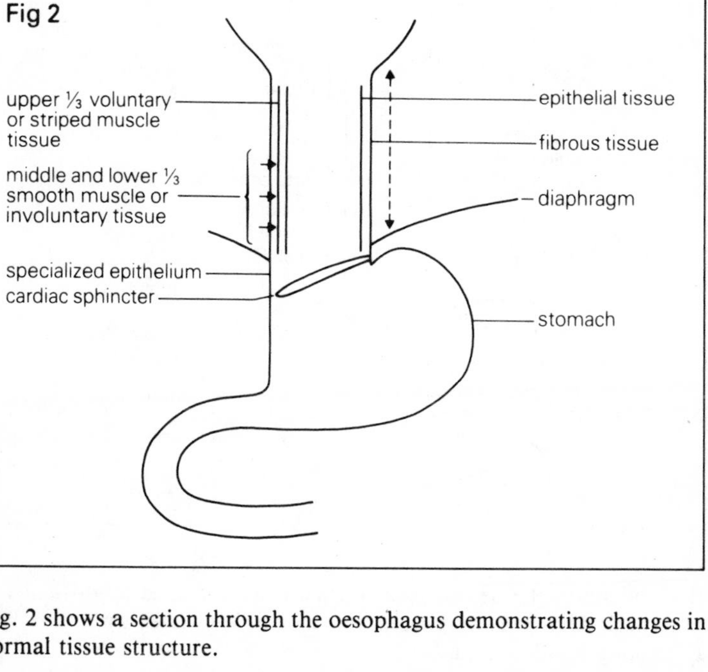

upper ⅓ voluntary or striped muscle tissue

middle and lower ⅓ smooth muscle or involuntary tissue

specialized epithelium
cardiac sphincter

epithelial tissue

fibrous tissue

diaphragm

stomach

Fig. 2 shows a section through the oesophagus demonstrating changes in normal tissue structure.

must be remembered and precautions must be taken to prevent it happening when **unconscious persons are in your care**.

2   The involuntary phase of swallowing happens in response to distention of the oesophagus by food. Aided by peristalsis and gravity, food passes downwards, the cardiac sphincter relaxes and food passes into the stomach. Hydrostatic pressure is higher in the oesophagus than in the stomach therefore gastric juices do not normally regurgitate into the oesophagus — (only when a person vomits), but in conditions such as **hiatus hernia** juices reflux from the stomach into the oesophagus causing inflammation and ulceration, eventually, causing **oesophagitis**. Many disease processes or lesions occur in the oesophagus.

Fig 3 shows a diagrammatic representation of sites where lesions occur.

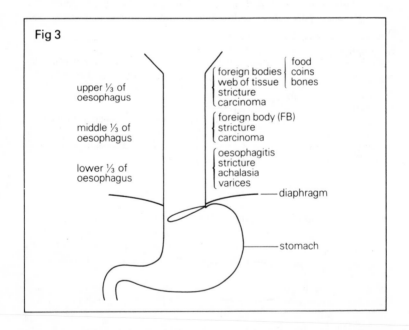

Fig 3

upper ⅓ of oesophagus

foreign bodies { food, coins, bones }
web of tissue
stricture
carcinoma

middle ⅓ of oesophagus

foreign body (FB)
stricture
carcinoma

lower ⅓ of oesophagus

oesophagitis
stricture
achalasia
varices

diaphragm

stomach

Dysfunction in the oesophagus is usually accompanied by difficulty in swallowing known as **dysphagia**, this may be associated with:

a   taking solids or liquids

b   iron deficiency, anaemia

in the lumen

c   obstruction in the wall   ⎱

outside the wall   ⎰

d   psychogenic illness

e   neuro muscular conditions

f   conditions of mouth or pharynx

From Table A, overleaf, compare and contrast the history, causative factors, problems experienced, investigations, treatments and surgical approaches that can be used for columns 1, 2, 3 and 4.

How could you meet the needs of patients suffering from these conditions? Make a plan.

As we have seen in Table A investigations specific to diagnosing diseases of the oesophagus are.

1   plain X-rays.

2   barium swallow/follow through

3   Oesophagoscopy and biopsy of tissue.

Patients who are to have these investigations must be given an explanation of the procedure in words they can understand (don't use technicalities).

1   Requires no specific preparation.

2   Involves fasting overnight. The specific instructions issued by the radiography department must be followed.

   a   The patient is given a gown to wear and is taken to the department with all notes and X-rays.

   b   The patient is asked to cooperate during the procedure, therefore if a hearing aid is worn this should remain with the patient.

   c   The patient will be asked to drink barium sulphate, a radio opaque non-toxic substance. The structure and functioning of the oesophagus is examined during the drinking of the barium and X-rays are taken. The X-rays will be reported on by the radiologist and should be obtained for the next consultant ward round.

   d   when the examination is complete ask:

      i   whether further X-rays are needed, or if the patient may take a meal.

      ii   **the patient must be told** if he **may not** eat or drink if further X-rays are required.

   e   After barium studies it is possible that:

      i   the patient will pass white stools

      ii   the patient may be constipated.

TABLE A   SHOWS COMMON DISEASES AND CONDITIONS OF

	1. BENIGN STRICTURE	2. MALIGNANT STRICTURE CARCINOMA	3. ACHALASIA OR CARDIO-SPASM
History	Longer than a year	Less than a year	Longer than a year
Sex Incidence	More common in females over 40	More common in males in 40-70 age group	More common in females
Causative Factor if known	Commonly hiatus hernia or Plummer Vinsons syndrome. Benign tumours are rare	Carcinoma	Not known, but Auerbach's plexus is defective. Sphincter does not effectively relax
Problems Experienced	**Dysphagia** (a) liquids can be swallowed (b) food sticks (c) symptoms are **intermittent** (d) heart burn and regurgitation are worsened by being or lying flat (e) oesophagitis can occur (f) there is weight loss and anaemia	**Dysphagia** (a) difficulty in swallowing solids at start of meal, this eases during the meal (b) symptoms are **continuous** (c) may soon be unable to swallow liquids (d) there is excessive salivation and regurgitation of food and weight loss. Mode of spread of malignant cells is (a) by direct infiltration (b) by lymph drainage and nodes	**Dysphagia** (a) difficulty in swallowing solids and liquids is experienced (cold drinks can cause severe pain) (b) vomiting and weight loss with anaemia occurs (c) inhalation of food can occur at night from the dilated oesophagus causing cough and pneumonia (d) mega oesophagus occurs if condition is untreated
Specific Investigations	Plain X-ray, barium swallow. Oesophagoscopy. Blood picture.	Plain X-ray, Barium swallow and follow through. Biopsy of growth. Skeletal survey. Blood picture. Cytology	Plain X-ray, Barium swallow. Oesophagoscopy. Blood picture
Specific Treatment	Dilation of stricture via oesophagoscope, repeated dilations may be necessary. For dense strictures a new oesophagus may be constructed from intestine or plastic. The bowel has to be prepared with **sulphonamides** and **antibiotics.**	Depends on the stage i.e. I, II, III, IV **If operable** the tumour is resected and radio therapy given. **If inoperable** palliative treatment is given i.e. (a) radio therapy (b) implantation of a Souttar or Celestin tube or a gastrostomy may be performed.	Depends on the stage of condition. **Early** treatment involves dilation and insertion of Plummers bag to disrupt fibres from inside. **Later** treatment Hellers operation or myotomy
Surgical Approach	Oral, abdominal or trans-thoracic	Oral for oesophagoscopy, abdominal or trans-thoracic	Oral for oesophagoscopy, abdominal or trans-thoracic

THE OESOPHAGUS AND INVESTIGATIONS

4. OESOPHAGITIS	5. OESOPHAGEAL VARICES	6. INJURIES FOREIGN BODIES
May be short or long history	Longer than a year	Acute in onset
Either sex	Either sex. More common in older age group. Can occur in young children	All age groups both sexes
Reflux of gastric juices. May result from burns, infection, indwelling tubes	Portal hypertension, varicose veins occur in the oesophagus and in the stomach	Accidental or intentional swallowing of corrosive substances or foreign bodies, coins, teeth
Dysphagia is due to inflammation and ulceration (see column 1). If this condition is untreated strictures will occur and may occur if the condition is treated	Bleeding occurs if pressure in the veins increases or if the veins are traumatised. Bleeding may be slow or a sudden massive haemorrhage may occur	Fear, pain, dysphagia, shock depending on cause. If corrosives have been swallowed there may be acute respiratory problems
Plain X-ray, Barium swallow, oesophagoscopy, Blood picture	Liver function tests. Barium swallow, follow through, oesophagoscopy	Plain X-ray, oesophagoscopy
Depends on cause. See column 1. If trauma is the cause, treatment is of the cause.	For massive bleeding a Sengstaken tube is passed and blood is replaced i.v. Vit K is given and pituitrin. A porta caval shunt or lienorenal shunt can be done later. Trans-oesophageal ligation.	Depends on cause. Oesophagoscopy can be done to remove f.b.'s. Hydrocortisone i.v. fluids and antibiotics minimise effects of burns. Dilation comes later.
See column 1	Abdominal trans-thoracic	

The patient should be informed of these eventualities to prevent unnecessary anxiety. Many elderly people are extremely bowel conscious and are concerned about constipation of only one day duration.

3   Oesophagoscopy describes examination of the oesophagus with an oesophagoscope. Preparation as for general anaesthesia — see chapter 1. In the anaesthetic room the anaesthetist may spray the patient's pharynx with local anaesthetic. After the examination is complete no food or drink should be allowed until sensation returns or the patient could inhale food or fluids. The patient must be **told why** he is not allowed a meal. All reports of examinations should be filed in the patients case notes. Concise reports are made in the Kardex.

Preparation for oesophageal surgery

See general principles of pre-operative care **chapter 1**.

Specific pre-operative preparation should entail a careful explanation of the intended procedure and the date on which it will be performed to the patient and relatives if necessary. An informed patient may more easily cope with the immediate post-operative period. Tell the relatives when they may phone.

The following factors will influence the way the patient is prepared.

1   The general physical state is assessed with reference to state of hydration and nutrition, deficiencies must be corrected and infections treated.

2   The psychological well-being, doubts and anxieties must be discussed. There may be social problems that can be solved with the help of the medical social worker. The needs of the patient have to be assessed.

3   The anticipated surgical approach. See Table A.

Post-operative general principles **See chapter 1**

Specific post-operative care after surgery is influenced by

1   the patient's physical state

2   his reaction to the operation.

It is difficult to lay down hard and fast rules as individuals should be independently assessed, reactions vary to similar operative procedures. Patients have to be helped to cope with wounds, drainage, restricted mobility, pain, fear, unaccustomed dependency, naso-gastric tubes and aspiration, intravenous infusions, c.v.p. lines, etc. A well informed patient may tolerate the immediate post-operative discomfort and may cooperate more readily with painful moving, coughing and deep breathing, thereby minimising the occurrence of preventable risks post-operatively and thus achievable goals may be set.

The immediate priorities are:

1   to maintain respiration and
2   circulation.

These priorities involve intelligent assessment of:

a   recovery from anaesthesia
b   colour
c   pulse rate and volume and temperature
d   blood pressure and respiratory rate and character
e   drainage and wound dressings.

Any deviation from normal expectations must be reported to the nurse in charge. If you are in doubt always ask a senior nurse to check your findings.

As soon as the patient's condition allows and he is able to cooperate he should be sat up gradually and be encouraged to move and breathe deeply.

Attention should be given to general hygiene including changes of bed linen and gowns. Urine passed should be recorded.

Relief of pain

Analgesics should be given as ordered. Expectations of tolerance to pain or value judgements concerning administration of pain relieving drugs **should not be made** as each individual reacts according to the level of his pain threshold, or his personality or culture and should be individually assessed. Expressions of fear or anxiety, pallor, sweating, flushing, a fast pulse, or restlessness may all indicate that analgesics are required. Some people are afraid to ask, or think they have to be stoical. It is important to remember that rest and sleep are paramount in helping the patient through the immediate recovery period. When a medication is to be given, follow the rules of administration of drugs laid down by your procedure committee. Assess the response of the patient to the analgesic, and if the pain is not relieved or if an adverse reaction is noted, the matter should be reported and noted in the Kardex.

Wounds and drainage

Wounds or the outer dressing and periphery should be observed for swelling and bleeding and the amount and character of drainage should be entered on the fluid balance chart. Remember that:

1   pain
2   tension round the wound, swelling and bruising

3   tachycardia with increasing rate and poor volume
4   increased and shallow respiratory rate — may indicate reactionary bleeding which can occur up to 48 hours post-operatively.

Report your findings, keep accurate records and do not alarm the patient.

Naso gastric aspiration

Rationale:
1   to keep the stomach empty
2   to prevent leakage from the anastomosis
3   to assess fluid lost from the G.I. tract

Naso gastric tubes may be drained by:

    a continuous or open drainage into a drainage bag. If this method is used, aspiration is still necessary at intervals.

    b Intermittent drainage. The naso gastric tube is spiggoted, and the stomach contents are aspirated at intervals.

        i   Observe the character and amount of fluid withdrawn.
        ii   Enter amount and character immediately on the fluid balance chart.
        iii Do not be too enthusiastic as over-suction can cause pain.
        iv   Any deviations from normal expectations should be reported.
        v   If no fluid is aspirated in the immediate post-operative period or should the patient become nauseated or vomit, steps should be taken to check the position and patency of the tube. It may be necessary to introduce a fresh tube.

Intravenous infusion

Intravenous therapy maintains the patient's fluid and electrolyte balance. The type of fluids infused depends on the patient's general state. The types of fluids used for short term therapy are:
1   Saline 0.9% w/v
2   Dextrose 5% w/v
3   Dextrose 4.0% w/v with 0.18% sodium chloride w/v

While the patient is receiving intravenous infusion the following routine is usually adopted viz:

Blood is taken daily to estimate
    a Haemoglobin
    b Electrolytes

Normal values for electrolytes in plasma are:

			OLD Units	**SI Units**
1	Na	= Sodium	137–147 m Eq/litre	135–145 mmol/litre
2	K	= Potassium	4–5.5 m Eq/litre	3.6–5.0 mmol/litre
3	Cl	= Chlorides	95–105 m Eq/litre	98–107 mmol/litre
4	HCO_3	= Bicarbonate	24–30 m Eq/litre	21–28 mmol/litre

The reports should be seen by the ward doctor daily and steps will be taken to correct electrolyte imbalance. All the pathology forms have lists of normal electrolyte values for comparison with the laboratory findings. If there is a serious deficiency, or excess, the person in charge should report the matter immediately.

Regime for caring for patients on short or long term therapy is listed below.

1 *General observations*
   a The skin should be warm, dry and the normal colour for the individual.
   b Vital signs should be within normal limits and recorded four-hourly.
   c Observe jugular venous pressure.
   d Test urine daily for specific gravity and chloride state particularly.
   e Difficulty in breathing or a cough must be reported as this may indicate oedema of the lungs from circulatory overloading.
   f Fluids given intravenously must be recorded by type and volume. Only prescribed and checked fluids may be given. If the container is damaged or the fluid cloudy do not use but return to the dispensary immediately. Check the following with a trained nurse:
      i   the prescription
      ii   the fluid
      iii the patient's identity
      iv   the rate of flow of fluid i.e. is to be infused in 6 or 8 hours.
      Also, keep accurate records of the fluid balance.
   g If the fluid is not infusing to time do **not** run through quickly to keep the schedule.

For long term intravenous therapy:
Patients receiving therapy over a long period of time should be given i.v. vitamins. The nutritional state can be maintained by giving intravenous fats, carbohydrates and proteins. Weight should be recorded as there is usually weight loss.

2   *Local observations*
   a The site of injection must be inspected. Swelling, pain or inflammation should be reported.
   b The rate of flow should be checked by counting the number of drips into the drip chamber in one minute. Approximately 17 drops/minute should be correct timing for 1 litre of fluid to be infused in 8 hours.
   c Raising the limb and keeping the area warm may help if a vein does go into spasm.
   d If a drip stops try to restart it, but **do not** inject any fluid through the needle, report the matter.
   e Should the needle become displaced the fluid will run into the tissues causing swelling. Slow down the drip and report the matter.
   f Examine fingers and/or calves for swelling.
   g Swelling can be caused by tight bandages.
   h Make sure the splint is comfortable.

Blood transfusion

Blood transfusions are given:
1   to restore blood volume
2   to correct anaemia.

Two people, one a trained nurse or doctor, must check the following with the patient's notes before setting up a blood transfusion.
1   The patients name, age and address (check with the wrist band and with the patient if possible).
2   The A.B.O. blood group.
3   The Rhesus factor.
4   The serial number and date.

All details should correspond with the patient's notes.
Blood should not be collected from the blood bank until needed. The blood is checked on collection from the blood bank and signed for.
Complications of blood transfusions may be:
1   A simple reaction to a foreign protein (the donor blood). There may be a transient rise in temperature, headache and increase in pulse rate.
     Action taken: the matter is reported and the transfusion slowed. The reaction of the patient is observed.
2   An allergic reaction is caused by allergy to foreign proteins. There may be headache, nausea, and an allergic urticarial rash. Action

taken: the drip is slowed and the matter reported. Usually piriton or other antihistamines are prescribed and the patient is observed.

3 Incompatibility occurs as a result of mismatch of the A.B.O. or Rhesus factor in the blood transfusion. Any patient receiving blood who

a has a rigor

b complains of severe pain in the loin

c has reduced urinary output — oliguria — with haemoglobinurea must have the transfusion stopped. The laboratory is informed and the donor blood is checked. There may have been a mistake in cross matching or if the procedure for checking blood was not closely adhered to, blood could have been given to the wrong patient. Air embolism is not so much of a risk these days with plastic floats and collapsible bags. If it occurs it is a serious complication.

Thrombophlebitis causes pain and inflammation in the infected vein. The infusion is stopped, the needle removed and reinserted elsewhere. The affected area is supported and rested. Right ventricular failure can occur if the patient is a poor risk. For poor risk patients the central venous pressure is measured. A rise in C.V.P. should be reported and the drip slowed.

d The same local and general observations given for intravenous therapy apply for blood transfusion and the T.P.R. B/P are taken hourly during transfusion and 4 hourly for 48 hours when transfusion is discontinued. Return all blood bags to the laboratory in a sealed container and take precautions when handling blood. Wash your hands, take care not to prick your skin, if you do so report the matter as there is a danger of hepatitis. Any reaction e.g. jaundice after the blood transfusion must be reported.

e Urine is tested for protein.

f The patient's needs must be catered for during intravenous infusion.

Tubes and drainage

Following a trans-thoracic approach for surgery (see Table A) an underwater seal drainage will be placed in the patient's chest. The patient should have been informed pre-operatively why his mobility will be restricted in relation to the chest tubes.

The principle of chest drainage is to restore natural lung function as soon as possible.

1   To extract air and fluid secretions from the chest cavity.
2   To prevent air entering the chest cavity through the wound.

The apparatus used must be checked carefully.
1   All tubes, connections, drainage bottles or bags must be securely connected. When the patient is to change his position the chest tubes must be clamped in two places, the clamps are removed immediately a comfortable position is assumed.
2   The drainage must be seen to function efficiently.
   a On breathing out, bubbles appear in the water seal.
   b On breathing in, the fluid in the underwater tube should move up the tube slightly.
   c If no activity on breathing is seen in the seal in the immediate post-operative period.
      i   Make sure the chest tubes are not clamped.
      ii The patient is not sitting or lying on the tubes. Action: try gently moving the tube. If the tube is patent and in position, **a** and **b** should be seen to occur. Inactivity should be reported immediately.
   d The type and amount of drainage should be observed and measured.
   e The patient's colour, respiratory rate, pulse rate and blood pressure should be checked frequently. Deviation from the normal should be reported.
   f An airtight dressing should be readily available in case of accidental removal of tube, this should be applied immediately over the stab wound and the matter reported.
   g All staff involved with the patient should understand the management of underwater seal drainage. Cleaners should not be allowed to move the bottles or bags.

Removal of chest drainage tubes
1   Apical and basal catheters are removed when normal lung function is restored. Activity in the underwater seal stops. An x-ray is taken and the doctor advises when the tube is to be removed.
    Chest tubes have two sutures to be dealt with:
   a a stay suture securing the tube to the skin
   b a purse string suture securing the stab wound edges.
Care must be taken to cut **only** the stay suture. The chest tube is clamped, the patient is asked to breath in, the tube is removed, the purse string is tied and an airtight dressing is applied.

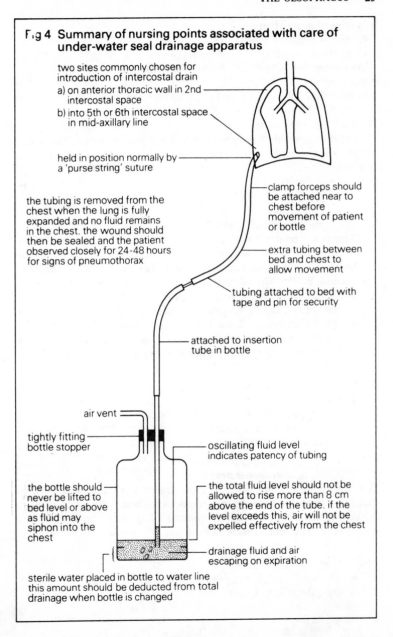

Fig 4 Summary of nursing points associated with care of under-water seal drainage apparatus

two sites commonly chosen for introduction of intercostal drain
a) on anterior thoracic wall in 2nd intercostal space
b) into 5th or 6th intercostal space in mid-axillary line

held in position normally by a 'purse string' suture

clamp forceps should be attached near to chest before movement of patient or bottle

extra tubing between bed and chest to allow movement

the tubing is removed from the chest when the lung is fully expanded and no fluid remains in the chest. the wound should then be sealed and the patient observed closely for 24-48 hours for signs of pneumothorax

tubing attached to bed with tape and pin for security

attached to insertion tube in bottle

air vent

tightly fitting bottle stopper

oscillating fluid level indicates patency of tubing

the bottle should never be lifted to bed level or above as fluid may siphon into the chest

the total fluid level should not be allowed to rise more than 8 cm above the end of the tube. if the level exceeds this, air will not be expelled effectively from the chest

drainage fluid and air escaping on expiration

sterile water placed in bottle to water line this amount should be deducted from total drainage when bottle is changed

It is important to observe:

colour — cyanosis must be reported.

respiration — dyspnoea must be reported.

movement of chest — both sides of the chest must move simultaneously.

Any deviation from the normal must be reported immediately.

Wound drainage tubes

Wound drainage tubes are removed when drainage ceases. The doctor advises when the tubes may be removed. There are two types of drains commonly used.

1 Redivac drains.
2 Corrugated drains.

1 *Principles of redivac drains*

This is a tube drain with perforations along its length. The redivac drain is laid in the wound at surgery and the end is brought out through a stab wound secured with a stay stitch and attached to a vacuum bottle. The advantage of this type of drainage is:

a the character of drainage can easily be seen
b the volume can be accurately measured in the bottle
c the bottles are sterilised after use and re-used. The antennae on the bottles indicate when the bottle should be changed, i.e. the bottle needs re-charging when the antennae meet together.

Removal of Redivac drains

a cut the stay suture
b clamp the tube and disconnect from the bottle
c apply firm traction to the tube and remove completely
d apply a small dressing to the stab wound.

2 *Principle of corrugated drains*

Corrugated drains may be rubber or plastic. They are usually laid in superficial tissues at surgery, the secretions run along the corrugations to the skin where a plastic bag, i.e. colostomy bag can be applied over the stab wound. The tube is secured by a stay stitch and a safety pin.

Removal of corrugated drains

a The stay stitch is removed
b the tube is withdrawn $\frac{1}{2}''$

c a fresh, sterile, safety pin is inserted near the skin and the excess drain is cut off. This procedure is repeated until the drain is removed completely.

All drainage must be recorded. The removal of drains is recorded into Kardex together with the state of the wound and general condition of the patient.

Gastrostomy

A tube is inserted via the anterior abdominal wall into the stomach. The purpose of this procedure is to maintain nutrition when there is an obstruction or inoperable carcinoma of the oesophagus through which a celestin type tube cannot be passed. In the latter situation the procedure is permanent, in the former situation the procedure may be temporary as preparation for reconstruction of the oesophagus.

The patient and relatives must be given a full explanation of the intended surgery. If a person understands the rationale of the procedure he may more easily come to terms with his problem. Specific care of a patient with a gastrostomy entails the following four principles.

1 To help the patient over the immediate post-operative phase.
2 To provide psychological and social support.
3 To observe principles of tube feeding:

   a Protection of the skin with a barrier cream is necessary as gastric juices will excoriate the skin and cause pain.
   b Fluids should be given through a funnel attached to the tube.
   c Calorific value of foods should be planned.
   d Records of food and fluids must be accurately kept.
   e Encourage the patient to be interested in his meals.
   f Remember that meal times are social occasions, and have conversations with the patient during feeds.
   g Observe reaction to meals:
      i diarrhoea can be caused by a diet too rich in fats and carbohydrates
      ii abdominal distension must be reported.
4 To provide follow up support when/if the patient is discharged from hospital.

Wound care

There is no need to inspect clean wounds, this could lead to wound infection. If the patient complains of pain or discomfort or if there is a rise in temperature or discharge seen, the wound should be inspected.

The doctor advises when sutures or clips are to be removed. Clips are usually removed from chest or abdomen about the 5th or 6th day. Sutures may be

1 continuous
2 interrupted
3 deep tension
4 subcutaneous.

Sutures are removed according to the surgeons preference. Alternate interrupted sutures are usually removed about the seventh day starting with the 2nd suture and ending with the penultimate suture. If all is well the remaining sutures are removed on the 9th or 10th day. Continuous sutures are removed about the 14th day post-operatively. The wound is inspected carefully. If there is a discharge a swab is taken and sent to the laboratory for culture and sensitivity.

For total basic principles of post-operative care see **chapter 1**. As soon as possible post-operatively, patients are encouraged to be independent. Their progress is carefully monitored and their needs assessed. When the time comes for discharge the following procedure is necessary:

1 Ascertain that their home environment is suitable for discharge. It may be necessary to send the patient to a convalescent hospital.
2 Inform the G.P. of the findings, date of discharge and follow-up treatment.
3 It may be necessary to have the district sister visit the patient in hospital to familiarise herself with the treatment.
4 An appointment is made for an out-patient visit and a card is supplied with the date and time of the appointment.
5 Order a seven day supply of drugs for the patient to take home if necessary and enclose a medication prescription sheet for the G.P.
6 Make sure the patient and/or his relatives understand the instructions given and the implications of his treatment.

Practice Questions

Test 1

Test your comprehension of this section of work by answering the following questions. You may find it necessary to re-read the section if you have several wrong answers.

1. Why are analgesics used?
2. What does benign mean?
3. Define the meaning of biopsy.
4. What does the term carcinoma describe?
5. What are Celestin and Souttar tubes used for?
6. What does Hiatus mean?
7. What does the word lesion describe?
8. Define the meaning of Hiatus Hernia.
9. What does the term palliative mean?
10. Give a definition of inflammation.
11. When are Sengstaken tubes used?
12. What does trauma mean?
13. Define thrombosphlebitis.
14. What does dysphagia describe?
15. What does resection mean?
16. What does anastamosis mean?
17. What does the word reflux describe?
18. Why are stay sutures used?
19. When are liver function tests performed?
20. What is the pathology of Myasthemia Gravis?
21. What drugs are used to sterilise the bowel pre-operatively?
22. Why is Vitamin K_1 given?
23. Why do oesophageal varices occur?
24. What does cytology mean?
25. What does myotomy mean?
26. Benign strictures in the oesophagus are more common in males than females? True/False?
27. Plummer Vinsons Syndrome is Synonymous with Patterson Kelly Brown Syndrome? True/False?
28. Achalasia is synonymous with cardiospasm? True/False?
29. Mediastinitis can occur after oesophagoscopy? True/False?

30. Which of the following investigations may be performed to diagnose diseases of the oesophagus?
    a Hypopharyngoscopy.
    b Barium meal.
    c Barium Swallow.
    d Cytology.
    e Biopsy.
31. Which one of the following is the primary cause of Oesophageal Varices?
    a Reflux Oesophagitis.
    b Hiatus Hernia.
    c Portal Hypertension.
    d Malignant Hypertension.
32. Which of the following symptoms occur in malignant disease of the oesophagus?
    a Cold drinks cause pain.
    b Food is regurgitated at night.
    c Symptoms are intermittent.
    d Symptoms are continuous.
    e Food sticks, fluid passes easily.
    f Liquids pass easily, food sticks.
33. Mrs. Davies a 55 year old housewife is admitted with a diagnosis of cirrhosis of the liver. On admission she is pale, cold and clammy.
    1. Which one of the following actions would you take?
        a   Give her a warm drink.
        b   Ask her if she is frightened.
        c   Put her into a warm bed.
        d   Check her pulse rate and blood pressure.
    2. Which of the following should be prepared in the event of severe bleeding occurring from oesophageal varices?
        a   A naso Gastric tube.
        b   A Celestin tube.
        c   A Sengstaken tube.
        d   A Souttar tube.
        e   An Endotracheal tube.
    3. Which of the following alterations in vital signs should be reported immediately?
        a   A rise in temperature.
        b   A drop in pulse rate.
        c   A drop in systolic and diastolic blood pressure.
        d   A dry, cold and pale skin.

4. Which of the following drugs may be given to lower portal blood pressure?
   a   Pitocin.
   b   Pituitrin.
   c   Pethedine.
   d   Pethilorfan.
34. You are in charge of a medical ward on intake. You are informed that a female patient with bleeding oesophageal varices is to be admitted.
   a   State how you would prepare for her admission. (30%)
   b   Describe the role of the nurse in the case of the patient and the probable lines of medical management. (55%)
   c   How would you explain the condition to a junior nurse? (15%)

Answers to Test 1

1. Analgesics, e.g. morphine sulphate, pethedine are used to relieve pain and sedate the patient.
2. The term benign used in relation to pathology means non-malignant.
3. The term biopsy means the removal of a small piece of living tissue for examination under the microscope, this is an aid to diagnosis.
4. The term carcinoma describes a type of cancer of epithelial cells. A malignant condition.
5. Celestin or Souttar tubes are inserted into the oesophagus. Gastrostomy is performed and the fine end of the tube is pulled through the cardiac sphincter into the stomach so that a patient with dense strictures or inoperable carcinoma of the oesophagus may take meals normally. This is a palliative procedure.
6. Hiatus means gap or opening.
7. A morbid or pathological change in an organ.
8. Hiatus hernia describes herniation or prolapse of part of the stomach through the oesophageal hiatus into the chest. Hiatus hernae are described as i) sliding, ii) rolling.
9. Palliative means treatment which relieves a condition but does not cure the condition.
10. Inflammation is the response of tissues to injury. The response is (a) swelling, (b) redness and heat, (c) loss of function, (d) pain.
11. Sengstaken tubes are used to control bleeding from oesophageal or gastric varices.
12. Trauma means injury.
13. Thrombophlebitis describes inflammation of veins.
14. Dysphagia describes difficulty in swallowing.

15. Complete removal of a diseased section, e.g. of stomach or intestine.
16. Anastomosis means either the establishment of an artificial join e.g. between two parts of the intestine, or the intercommunication of the terminal branches of two or more blood vessels.
17. The flow of gastric juices from the stomach into the oesophagus.
18. To secure drainage tubes to the skin most commonly, though during operation they are used to support tissue out of the surgeon's way.
19. During investigation of diseases of the liver, gall bladder, etc.
20. Weakness of muscular activity (neuro muscular dysfunction) associated with a deficiency of acetylcholine and excessive cholinesterase causing failure of transmission of nerve impulses in the motor end plate.
21. Sulphonamides, antibiotics, nystatin.
22. To increase clotting power.
23. Back pressure on the portal vein.
24. Examination or study of cells.
25. Cutting through a muscle or division of muscle fibres.
26. False, there is a higher incidence among females.
27. True.
28. True.   31. c.   33. 2. c
29. True.   32. d.e.   33. 3. c
30. c.d.e.   33. 1. d   33. 4. b

Model Answer to question 34

a Includes planning and management of resources.
    Delegate staff to prepare
    a an admission bed easily accessible for the night staff.
    b Check that O_2 and suction are available and in working order. Several suction bottles will be necessary.
    c Bed elevator and drip stands are assembled.
    d Blood transfusion trolley is prepared. Vene section or cut down may be necessary.
    e Naso-gastric tray with Sengstaken tube.
    f Charts, vomit bowls, paper towels, mouth wash.
    g Thermometer and sphygmomanometer. It may be necessary to obtain a sphygmomanometer from the recovery room so that you do not distress or disturb the patient unnecessarily, i.e. (special type).
    h Inform your nursing officer that the patient is arriving, it will be necessary to have access to the dangerous drugs cupboard.

b On admission the patient is put into bed. Inform the doctor and make an immediate nursing assessment. Make the patient as comfortable as possible, reassure her. If the patient is bleeding the first priority is to arrest bleeding. Blood vomited should be measured and recorded on fluid balance chart. Delegate a person to take a history from the relatives.

Medical management will include an immediate assessment of condition.

  i A Sengstaken tube can be passed orally, the balloons on the tube are inflated to apply pressure to oesophageal or gastric varices in an attempt to stop the bleeding.

  ii Blood is taken for grouping and cross matching and packed cell volume, full blood count and prothrombin time.

  iii An intravenous infusion is commenced until blood is ready for transfusion.

  iv Drugs may be given to relieve anxiety and to constrict blood vessels.

  v The immediate aim is to stop bleeding and restore blood volume.

  vi It may be necessary to take the patient to theatre for ligation of the bleeding veins.

  vii The long term aim is a) to investigate the cause of the varices b) treat the cause if possible (c) porto caval shunt may be done.

A nursing assessment should be made of the patient's physical and mental state, and a regime of care prescribed. Reassurance, explanation and co-operation of the patient are vital as are care of: i.v.i., see previous notes; for **aspiration,** see previous notes; specific care of Sengstaken tube — balloons must be deflated for 5 minutes in each hour so that oesophageal or gastric mucus membrane is not damaged; fluid balance chart should be kept accurately; urine is tested and vital signs recorded; general reaction and mobility of the patient noted and physical movement encouraged. Talk to the patient. Good communication is essential so that unnecessary anxiety may be avoided.

c Oesophageal varices occurr from pressure on the portal vein, cirrhosis of the liver is a common cause, though there are other causes, i.e. congenital abnormalities. Pressure on the portal vein eventually causes veins in the lower end of the oesophagus to dilate, gastric veins may also dilate. Trauma to these veins or increased intra abdominal pressure may cause bleeding which may be slow, or there may be a massive haemorrhage.

3 REGIONAL AND APPLIED STRUCTURE AND FUNCTION OF THE STOMACH AND DUODENUM

Fig. 5 shows a diagrammatic representation of the stomach, duodenum, liver, gallbladder, pancreas and spleen. Revise with textbook models and your lecture notes. Learn to draw line diagrams and label them correctly. Practice makes perfect.

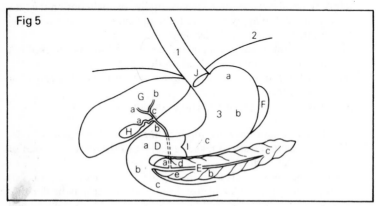

Fig 5

Key

1 oesophagus

2 diaphragm

3 stomach   a fundus b body   c pyloric antrum

D duodenum   a 1st   b 2nd   c 3rd parts

E pancreas   a head   b body   c tail
                   d common bile duct   e pancreatic duct
                   f ampulla of Vata

F spleen

G liver   a and b Rt. + Lt. hepatic ducts
         c common hepatic ducts

H gallbladder   a cystic duct   b common bile duct

I pyloric sphincter

J cardiac sphincter

Refer to anatomical models for relationship with abdominal walls, vertebrae, kidneys, colon, aorta, vena cava, nerves and lymphatics.
Fig. 6 Shows a diagrammatic representation of tissues, cells and acid and alkaline areas of the stomach.

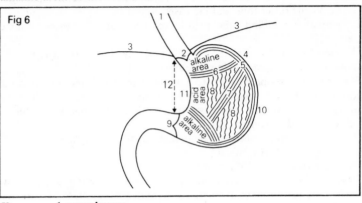

Key

1 oesophagus
2 cardiac sphincter
  concerned with preventing reflux
  of gastric juice
3 diaphragm
4 outer peritoneal coat protective — prevents friction

muscle fibres
  5 outer longitudinal   concerned with gastric motility,
  6 middle circular   peristalsis and with gastric juice
  7 inner oblique   reduces food to chyme.

mucus membrane
  8 Inner lining is thrown into folds or
    rougae and contains gastric glands
    which secrete gastric juice containing:

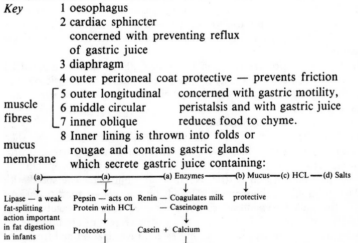

9 pyloric sphincter concerned with preventing reflux of chyme
10 greater curvature of stomach
11 lesser curvature of stomach
12 acid area with parietal and oxyntic cells
   secreting acid pepsin and mucous

Ulcers usually occur on the lesser curvature of the stomach. Ulcers occurring on or near the pylorus or cardia have a higher incidence of malignancy.

Nerve supply of the stomach is 1. Parasympathetic and 2. Sympathetic.

1. The Vagus raises tone and increases peristalsis.

2. Sympathetic inhibits the pyloric sphincter and increases alkaline secretion.

The blood supply is mediated via: 3. the R. and L. gastric arteries

4. the R. and L. gastro epiploic arteries

There are corresponding veins to 3 and 4. The tributories drain into the portal vein. Lymph vessels accompany blood vessels and drain into the aortic, gastric, splenic and mesenteric nodes, an important factor in indirect spread of cancer cells.

Gastric secretion is controlled by two mechanisms, they are:

1. Nervous   2. Hormonal

There are three stages in the process.

Stage 1 in the process is called the **cephalic phase**, and is initiated by sight, smell, taste and thought of food. The **hypothalamus** sends out increased impulses to the vagus nerve supplying the stomach and the increased vagal activity stimulates oxyntic and parietal cells to produce gastric juice rich in acid + pepsin and the cells are made sensitive to the hormone **gastrin**.

Stage 2 in the process is called the **gastric phase**, and is initiated by increased vagal activity and by the pressure of food in the pyloric antrum. A hormone called gastrin is released, it circulates in the blood stream and sustains the activity of gastric cells.

Stages 1 and 2 are interdependent.

Stage 3 in the process is called the *intestinal phase*, and is initiated when food reaches the intestine, here a hormone called enterogastrone is produced, because of the action of enterogastrone fatty meals are slow to leave the stomach and gastric secretions are inhibited. The speed with which food leaves the stomach depends on the type of food taken. An operation called a vagotomy can be performed to reduce vagal activity, therefore motility of the stomach and gastric secretions are inhibited.

Compare and contrast the cause and effect, investigation and treatment of diseases of the stomach described in Table B on p. 38

Individuals need surgical intervention when:

1 medical treatment fails

2 complications arise

3 the patient cannot work.

The main reasons for emergency admission to hospital are:

1 Perforation of peptic ulcer (see signs symptoms and lines of treatment in Table B)
2 Haematemesis and melaena. Emergency treatment is performed if:
   a bleeding continues
   b bleeding re-occurs
   c the patient is over 50 years when arteriosclerotic changes may indicate early surgery.

Vital signs to be observed if a patient is bleeding are as follows.
It is important to keep accurate records and report changes.

	A Signs indicating bleeding	**B** Signs indicating bleeding is stopping
Pulse	Tachycardia with poor volume	Rate slows, volume improves
Skin	Pale cold and clammy to touch	Colour improves, feels warm
B/P	Low systolic and diastolic pressure	B/P rises (watch carefully as bleeding can occur at this time)
Respirations	Rapid — there may be gasping	Slows to normal
General State	May experience fainting and weakness, may not be able to see clearly. May be apprehensive and be in pain. Some patients say they have a salty taste in the mouth and pass melaena stools.	Begins to feel better and look better

If signs listed in column **A** are observed, report should be made to the person in charge, the following steps are taken.

1 Reassure and rest the patient.
2 Raising the foot end of the bed helps relieve fainting.
3 Give morphia if prescribed.
4 In some centres a naso-gastric tube is passed and the blood is aspirated.

TABLE B COMMON DISEASES OF THE STOMACH &
(Congenital conditions are omitted)

| | Peptic Ulcers | |
	Gastric Ulcer (1)	Duodenal Ulcer (2)
History	Peptic Ulcers may be acute or chronic & co-exist	
	There may be a family history. There is usually a long history of complaints	There is usually a family history. There is usually a long history of complaints 5-10 times more common than G.U.
Sex Incidence	Incidence higher in males 40 years +	Incidence higher in males 25-50 year age group.
Predisposing Factors	Acute ulceration of stomach & duodenum may result from burns or drug(s). Chronic peptic ulcers more commonly seen than acute ulcers.	
	Chronic G.U. cause unknown. Incidence higher in manual worker group. There may be an association with smoking. No precise proof of relationship with blood group. Secretion of H.C.L. normal or low.	Chronic D.U. cause unknown. Incidence higher in professional group. There may be an association with smoking and stress. More common in people with blood group O. Secretion of H.C.L. is high in acid and pepsin.
S & S or Problems Experienced	**Periodicity** exacerbations lasting 2-6 weeks; followed by remissions of 2-6 months in Spring and Autumn. **Pain** is epigastric, occurs soon after a meal, but not usually at night. **Relieved** by vomiting, lying down, alkalis. **Appetite** is poor. Self-restricting diet imposed. **Weight** reduces.	**Periodicity** exacerbation lasting 2-6 weeks followed by remission of 2-6 months. Attacks common in Spring and Autumn. **Pain** severe & epigastric, occurs commonly in the night 2/3 hours after a meal — hunger pain. **Relieved** by eating, self induced vomiting, alkalis. **Appetite** is good, eats most foods. **Weight** maintains or increases.
Specific Investigations	Plain X-ray, stool studies G.F.T. Barium studies Gastrostomy or Fibroscopy	See Col. 1. Possible duodenal biopsy.
Complications	Loss of work Pyloric Stenosis Haematemises Perforation Melaena Malignancy	See Col. 1. Never becomes malignant.
Treatment Surgical Approach	Medical treatment tried initially.	
	Abdominal Partial gastrectomy is usually performed. Bilroth I to remove ulcer bearing area.	**Abdominal** Partial gastrectomy polya type to remove ulcer bearing area or vagotomy and pyloroplasty or antorectomy, occasionally gastro-enterostomy is performed.

DUODENUM INVESTIGATION & TREATMENT

Acquired Pyloric Stenosis (3)	Carcinoma of Stomach (4)	Perforation of Stomach or Duodenum (5)
Long history of complaints of stomach disorder. In women onset may be slow and silent.	Insidious	Acute in onset.
Either sex	Incidence higher in males 40-70 year group	Incidence higher in males
(1) Peptic ulcers causing scarring by fibrosis near the pylorus. (2) Carcinoma of stomach	(1) There may be an association with blood group A. (2) Individuals suffering from pernicious anaemia are 3 times more likely than non-sufferers to develop carcinoma.	Complication of peptic ulcer. There is: erosion of tissue mucosa — muscle & peritoneum, causing perforations, gastric or duodenal contents soil the abdominal cavity causing chemical irritation — peritonitis.
Periodicity is lost. **Pain** dyspepsia and fullness more evident in the evening, abdomen distention may be seen. **Relieved** by vomiting that is (i) Copious in volume and (ii) contains undigested food taken 1-2 days previously. **Weight** reduces.	**Periodicity** may be similar to peptic ulcer. **Pain** There may be no pain, only discomfort until secondaries are formed. There may be no symptoms until secondaries are established. Significant S & S (i) Weight loss (ii) Anorexia (iii) Malaise & weakness (iv) Vomiting (v) Lump may be obvious (vi) Lymph nodes palpable.	**Pain** Sudden & excruciating in the abdomen, may be referred to shoulder. Significant signs: (i) Rigid abdomen (ii) Vomiting only 1 × 2 (iii) Pulse rate initially slow (iv) Pallor, anxiety, reluctance to move (v) Shock.
See Col. 1.	See Col 1. + Skeletal Survey Possible Biopsy	Radiography on admission shows air bubble under diaphragm.
Dehydration. Tetany and Uraemia if untreated	Pyloric stenosis. Direct & Indirect spread of carcinoma.	Peritonitis. Subphrenic abscess.
Abdominal Partial gastrectomy or gastro enterostomy. Vagotomy & pyloroplasty may be done where D.U. is the cause.	**Abdominal** Total gastrectomy. The primary growth is removed where possible. Radiotherapy.	**Conservative** i.v.i. nasogastric tube. Analgesics and watch for improvement. **Surgical** Abdominal approach. (i) The perforation may be repaired with omentum or may be sutured. (ii) Vagotomy or pyloroplasty (iii) Partial gastrectomy can be performed.

TABLE C INVESTIGATIONS SPECIFIC TO THE STOMACH

	Barium Studies (1)	Gastric Function Tests (2)
Rationale involved	The principle of Barium studies has been explained in previous section.	G.F.T. are devised to measure the variations in volume and content of gastric juice.
Specific Tests	Barium meal & follow through, screening radiography of stomach & small intestine, diagnostic techniques where peptic ulcers, pyloric stenosis or gastric carcinoma is suspected.	Diagnostic techniques used to investigate suspected peptic ulcers, pyloric stenosis, gastric carcinoma, pernicious anaemia. Tests commonly used are: (i) Augmented histamine (ii) Night juice test (iii) Diagnex blue (iv) Schilling test.
Preparation for the tests	The patient is given an aperient the previous night. Meals are omitted until the examination is complete. All X-rays and notes are sent to the radiography dept. together with the patient at the appointed time.	The patient fasts prior to the test. A naso-gastric tube is passed, testing juice is removed and labelled. The stimulant is given and the routine for the test is followed. For tests (iii) and (iv) an N.G. tube is not passed and urine is collected after the stimulants have been administered.
Positive results to the tests	**Gastric Ulcers** show as a crater which fills with barium, and retains barium for some time after. **Duodenal Ulcers** (i) Deform the duodenal cap. (ii) The stomach empties quickly. (iii) A crater may be seen. **Pyloric Stenosis** causes delayed emptying of the stomach. **Long Standing Ulcers** may alter the shape of the stomach — hour-glass appearance. **Carcinoma** may show an irregular outline with filling defect.	**Achlorhydria** means the stomach cannot produce gastric juice with a pH of less than 7.1. The stomach does not respond to histamine stimulation. Seen in: (i) Pernicious anaemia (ii) Gastric carcinoma (iii) Post long-standing gastrectomy. **Hyperchlorhydria** means there is a high acid content, occurs commonly in duodenal ulcer when acid & pepsin content is high. In gastric ulcer there may be a variation between normal and higher than normal secretion.
After Care	As stated in previous section on Barium Studies.	Adverse reaction to stimulants should be watched for, i.e. hypotension.

& DUODENUM ARE AS FOLLOWS

Endoscopy (3)	Stool Studies (4)	Blood Studies (5)
Examinations devised to inspect the interior of the stomach and duodenum.	Tests devised to analyse whether occult or hidden blood is being passed in the stools.	Tests on venous blood to estimate whether the Hb and blood count is within normal limits.
Diagnostic techniques used are: (i) Gastroscopy (ii) Fibroscopy (iii) Gastric camera	Diagnostic techniques are: (i) Three day stools collected for laboratory analysis (ii) Haematest done in the ward, using amestest tablets.	Diagnostic technique to establish if the patient is suffering with anaemia.
The patient fasts overnight. The tests are usually done under local anaesthetic. It may be necessary to wash out the stomach prior to the tests.	(i) The patient abstains from eating meat for three days prior to tests (ii) and avoids vigorous brushing of teeth, a specimen of stool is collected on 4th, 5th & 6th day for laboratory analyses. (iii) For haematest follow manufacturers instructions.	No preparation necessary.
Peptic ulcers may be seen on visual examination which may not appear on radiography, or it may be necessary to differentiate between ulcers and carcinoma.	A positive result on either test means that bleeding which is not apparent to the naked eye is occuring. These tests are of value in (i) Diagnosis of peptic ulcers. (ii) Monitoring whether ulcers have healed. (iii) Continuous bleeding may indicate carcinoma.	Haemoglobin levels are reduced in anaemia. Red cell numbers are decreased in anaemia. The appearance of red cells is small in iron deficiency anaemia, large in pernicious anameia. The E.S.R. may be raised.
The patient is to fast until sensation returns to pharynx. Sore throats may be eased by gargles.	Observe stools for melaena. Black tarry offensive stools.	Observe puncture site for bleeding.

Intelligent nursing can allay collapse. Remember that a small amount of blood loss is frightening to the patient and his relatives, be calm and reassuring.

The principles of medical treatment in severe bleeding from the stomach are to:

1   sedate the patient
2   replace blood lost
3   prevent avoidable complications.

See chapter 1 for general pre-operative care.

Specific pre-operative preparation for gastric surgery depends on the type of admission and the patient's general state of well-being.

The emergency patient may only have skin toilet and a naso-gastric tube inserted and an intravenous infusion as pre-operative preparation.

To have elective surgery the patient must be as fit as possible.

   a   Infections are treated.
   b   Nutrition is improved.
   c   Anaemia is corrected.
   d   Electrolyte and vitamin deficiencies are treated.
   e   For patients with pyloric stenosis the stomach is washed out for three days prior to the surgery. This procedure cleans and restores tone to the stomach.
   f   Patients will be prepared according to the surgeon's instructions.
   g   A naso-gastric tube is passed.
   h   An intravenous infusion is commenced.

See **Table B** for types of surgery to stomach and duodenum.

Fig. 7 (a,b,c,d) shows a series of diagrammatic representations of types of surgery that may be performed for stomach and duodenal disease. Learn to draw these outlines, it is useful for explaining procedures to junior nurses.

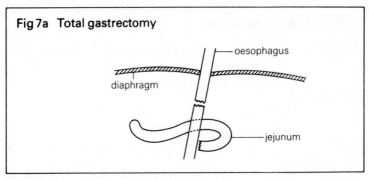

Fig 7a   Total gastrectomy

The stomach is removed. The oesophagus is joined or anastomosed to the jejunum — Roux-on-Y — a different route.

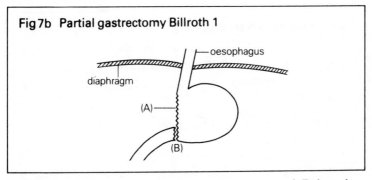

Fig 7b   Partial gastrectomy Billroth 1

The ulcer bearing part of the stomach **A** has been removed. **B** shows how continuity is restored.

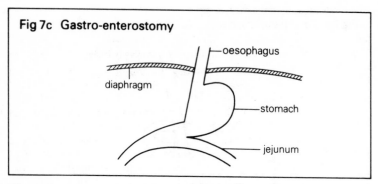

Fig 7c Gastro-enterostomy

The stomach is anastomosed to the jejunum.

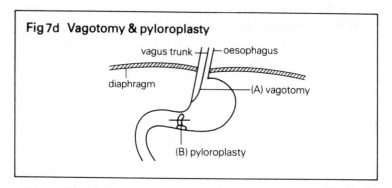

Fig 7d Vagotomy & pyloroplasty

A Selective vagotomy means that the branch of the vagus nerve supplying the stomach is divided.

B Pyloroplasty, the pyloric antrum is incised longitudinally and is resutured horizontally. Vagotomy slows the motility of the stomach. Pyloroplasty effects better drainage.

Post Operative Care Please refer to **basic principles in chapter 1** and to principles set out with reference to oesophageal surgery.

Specific Care after surgery of stomach and duodenum includes

1   Maintenance of circulation and respiration.
2   Gastric aspiration:
    a measure amount of aspirate

    b observe character of aspirate

    c record a + b on fluid balance chart.

3   Intravenous infusion

    a observe the limb site of infusion for i position, ii warmth, iii swelling, iv inflammation

    b Rate of flow — count drops per minute regulate according to orders. **Timing** is important.

    c Type of infusion in progress — check next prescription.

    d Additives must be checked with a responsible person and the prescription sheet. Ensure that additives are compatible with type of infusion i.e. lignocaine will precipitate out of Dextrose 5%, check compatibility chart. All additives must be mixed well in the solution. A label stating the type and amount of additive must be attached to the infusion bag. The response of the patient to the additives must be observed.

    e Keep accurate records

4   Check:

    a urinary output — test urine — record on fluid balance chart.

    b bowel sounds — when normal activity is returning 'gurgling' can be heard through the stethoscope.

    c drain's output should be measured and charted.

When bowel sounds are heard and naso-gastric aspirations diminish in volume, small amounts of fluid are given orally. Regime is usually:

1   30 mls of sterile water 2 hourly for 24 hours.

2   30 mls of water + milk 1 hourly for 24 hours.

3   If fluids are tolerated the naso-gastric tube is removed.

4   Increased amounts of fluids are given, if tolerated.

5   The intravenous infusion is removed.

Vomiting and abdominal distension should be watched for. If all is well, light diet is given, i.e. soups, ice cream and jelly to start, building up to minced meat, mashed vegetables, to normal diet before the patient leaves hospital. Following total partial gastrectomy, gastro-enterostomy, vagotomy and pyloroplasty it is advisable to take small meals and chew food well. It is possible for a food bolus to cause intestinal obstruction if the patient swallows whole segments of orange or whole pickled onions! Patients should be advised to take small meals and to rest after them. Post-operatively there may be mild dyspepsia, patients must be told of this pre-operatively otherwise they may be very disappointed in the result. Follow up treatment is important and an out-patient appointment must be made for fairly soon after discharge.

See advice given previously regarding discharge of patients from hospital.
Specific complications that can arise after gastrectomy or vagotomy and pyloroplasty are:

1. **Early complications**

   a   Haemorrhage $\begin{array}{l}\text{— Reactionary}\\ \text{— Secondary}\end{array}$

   b   Stomal obstruction

   c   Fistula

   d   Anastomotic ulcer

2. **Late complications**

   a   Dumping syndrome

   b   Hypoglycaemia

   c   Bilious vomiting

   d   Weight loss

   e   Diarrhoea

   f   Iron deficiency anaemia

   g   Malabsorption

Practice Questions

Test 2

Test your comprehension of this section of the work by answering the following questions. Answer all the questions in writing then check the answers. You may find it necessary to re-read the section if you have several answers wrong.

1. What does the term dumping syndrome mean?
2. When may hypoglycaemia occur?
3. What does malabsorption mean?
4. Define fistula.
5. What does arteriosclerosis mean?
6. Define the term anastomotic ulcer.
7. What does tachycardia mean?
8. Which of the following enzymes starts the chemical breakdown of protein in the stomach?
   a Renin
   b Lipase
   c Pepsin
   d Gastrin
9. Which one of the following examinations is performed to examine the stomach?
   a Oesophagoscopy
   b Peritoneoscopy
   c Fibroscopy
   d Hypopharyngoscopy
10. Which of the following statements regarding occurrence of pain associated with duodenal ulcers is correct? Pain occurs
    a Immediately after eating
    b A few hours after eating
    c Whilst a meal is taken
    d At no specific time.
11. Which of the following statements is correct regarding the temperature of fluid for gastric washout?
    a 100°C
    b 105°C
    c 40°C
    d 37°C

12. Which of the following statements is correct regarding sex incidence and social class in relation to occurrence of duodenal ulcer? Duodenal ulcer occurs commonly in men in:
   a Social Class 1 + 2
   b Social Class 4 + 5
   c Sex and Social Class is not an important factor.

13. Which of the following statements is correct regarding sex incidence and social class in relation to occurrence of gastric ulcer? Gastric ulcer occurs commonly in men in:
   a Social Class 1 + 2
   b Social Class 4 + 5
   c Sex and Social Class is not an important factor.

14. Which of the following statements regarding melaena stools is correct? Melaena stools are a sign of bleeding from:
   a Haemorrhoids
   b Peptic ulcers
   c Diverticulae
   d Perforated ulcer.

15. Which of the following statements regarding surgical treatment of gastric carcinoma is correct? Surgery for gastric carcinoma may be:
   a Vagotomy and pyloroplasty
   b Gastro-enterostomy
   c Total gastrectomy
   d Partial gastrectomy.

16. Which of the following statements is an important symptom of congenital pyloric stenosis?
   a Haematemesis
   b Abdominal distension
   c Pain
   d Projectile vomiting.

17. Which of the following statements regarding gastric lavage is correct? Excessive lavage using normal saline may induce:
   a Water intoxication
   b Electrolyte imbalance
   c Gastric irritation.

Complete the following sentences by placing one word in each space provided.

18. The stomach is covered externally by .*Peritoneal coat*

19. The tissue of the stomach lining is *mucosa*

20. The gastric hormone is called .*gastrin*

21. Gastric juice contains *HCl, pepsin, salt, mucus, intrinsic factor enzymes*

22. Enzymes in gastric juice are pepsin, rennin, lipase

23. The middle wall of the stomach is composed of muscle fibres, outer longitudinal middle circular inner oblique fibres.

24. The first part of the small intestine is the Duodenum

25. Match the investigations from **List II** below to the conditions in **List I**. Write the selected letter of your choice from **List II** against the condition in **List I**.

List I

1   Stomatitis
2   Haemorrhoids
3   Intestinal obstruction
4   Congenital pyloric stenosis
5   Gastro-enteritis
6   Cystic fibrosis

List II

A   Barium swallow
B   Swab for culture and sensitivity
C   Sigmoidoscopy
D   Liver function test
E   Plain X-ray
F   Chloride skin test
G   Stools for culture and sensitivity
H   Barium swallow
I   Barium enema
J   Gastro-graffin test

26. Select from **List II** the symptom which matches the disease in **List I**.

List I

1   Carcinoma of oesophagus
2   Portal hypertension
3   Perforated ulcer
4   High intestinal obstruction
5   Carcinoma of large intestine
6   Hiatus hernia
7   Pernicious anaemia

List II

A   Water brash
B   Glossitis
C   Haemorrhage
D   Melaena stools
E   Dysphagia
F   Gastritis

G   Effortless vomiting
H   Alternating diarrhoea and constipation
I   Rigid abdomen

27. Mr. Jones, a widower of 70 years, is admitted with a diagnosis of gastric carcinoma. He has been living alone since the death of his wife. On arrival on the ward he is thin, neglected in appearance and aggressive.

1. Which of the following actions would be most appropriate to take after Mr Jones has been admitted?
   a   Put him into bed
   b   Give him a bath and clean clothes
   c   Take and record his vital signs
   d   Sit and talk with him for a while

2. Which of the following is most important when Mr Jones is given a stomach washout?
   a   To keep the fluid hot
   b   To keep the fluid warm
   c   To use three litres of fluid
   d   To take the temperature of the fluid

3. Which of the following actions should the nurse take if on return to the ward after surgery the intravenous fluid is not running? Would you:
   a   Release the control valve
   b   Turn the control valve off
   c   Report the matter
   d   Examine the site of the needle

4. Which of the following should be reported immediately to the Ward Sister when recording Mr Jones' vital signs post operatively?
   a   A slow respiratory rate
   b   A low temperature
   c   Diastolic blood pressure of 60 mm Hg
   d   Systolic blood pressure of 60 mm Hg

5. Which of the following is the most important part of Mr Jones' post operative care?
   a   Skin hygiene
   b   Reassurance
   c   Oral toilet
   d   Exercising

28. Mrs Ford, a widowed lady of 60 years, has been admitted to hospital with a diagnosis of gastric ulcer. She is to have a partial gastrectomy performed.

a Describe the nurse's role in her pre-operative preparation   30%
b Describe the care that will be required for 48 hours following the operation   50%
c What advice should be given to Mrs Ford subsequent to her discharge?   20%

Answers to Test 2

1. Dumping syndrome may occur after gastrectomy. Food passes quickly into the small intestine and absorbs water from the circulation by osmosis, distension of the gut occurs, the patient sweats, has palpitations, fainting after meals is fairly typical.

2. Hypoglycaemia means there is a deficiency of sugar in the blood. This occurs sometimes when the patient fasts or if insulin is taken without food. The patient sweats, is giddy and has blurred vision. In diabetic persons hypoglycaemia is a serious condition. If the blood sugar is not raised the person may go into coma.

3. Malabsorption. Inability to absorb nutrition from the small intestine.

4. Fistulae are abnormal passages between the epithelial surfaces, e.g. fistula in ano.

5. Arteriosclerosis describes degeneration and hardening of arteries.

6. Anastomotic ulcer occurs on the artificial join of tissue or anastomosis e.g. in partial gastrectomy.

7. Tachycardia means a rapid pulse rate.

8. c   12. a   15. c
9. c   13. b   16. d
10. b   14. b   17. b
11. c

18. Peritoneum
19. Mucus membrane
20. Gastrin
21. Enzymes, mucous, HCL, Salts
22. Pepsin, Renin, Lipase
23. Muscle longitudinal, circular, oblique
24. Duodenum
25. 1 = B   2 = C   3 = E   4 = J   5 = G   6 = F
26. 1 = E   2 = C   3 = I   4 = G   5 = H   6 = A   7 = B
27. 1 = d   2 = d   3 = d   4 = d   5 = d

Model Answer to Question 28

a   A nursing assessment is made of Mrs Ford's mental and physical
state and her usual routine of sleep, diet, drugs taken, elimination,
effectiveness of hearing, social background. Elicit whether there are
any worries concerning hospitalisation in which the nursing or
medical staff, priest, family or medical worker can help. Carry out
efficiently prescribed treatment and investigation which may include
preparation for barium studies, gastric function tests, stomach
washouts, endoscopy and after care. Keep accurate records of pre-
operative events. Obtain laboratory test findings and X-rays. Ask
doctor to prescribe hypnotics if necessary, help doctor in
examination and setting up i.v.i. On the day of operation and
according to the laid-down hospital procedure, check that Mrs Ford
has:

i   fasted overnight
ii   emptied lower bowel
iii   removed dentures, clips, make-up, valuables
iv   taken a bath and been shaved
v   a wrist identity band properly filled in
vi   a naso-gastric tube inserted
vii   a gown and cap on
viii passed urine
ix   been given her premedication
x   been placed safely on the theatre trolley
xi   notes and X-ray complete for theatre

b   On return to the ward and while on the trolley check Mrs Ford's
general condition. Place her gently into bed, quickly examine the
wound dressing, drainage and i.v.i. Cover the patient with
bedclothes and if conscious put a pillow under her head, secure the
drainage bottle. Ascertain the i.v.i. is running efficiently, examine
the fingers for swelling and the bandage for tightness or wetness.
Take and record the vital signs and record, aspirate, the naso-gastric
tube and record character and amount of aspirate. Report
abnormalities immediately. Half-hourly observations of vital signs
will be necessary until the general condition is satisfactory. Gently
raise Mrs Ford into a sitting position, and encourage deep breathing,
coughing and leg movements as soon as she is able. Analgesics
should be given for pain and she should rest as much as possible.
Record when urine is passed and test the urine. If she feels nauseated
aspirate the naso-gastric tube. Offer mouth washes, help her to
move. Wash her as soon as she wants and give a cool gown to wear

so that she is comfortable. The frequency with which vital signs are taken and naso-gastric aspirations made, depends on her general condition. The timing of the regime of intravenous fluids should be adhered to.

The next day continue with the above routine, assess Mrs Ford's general condition, check tubes and drainage of i.v.i. limb, change redivac bottles, check fluid balance chart and check dressing of wound. Help the doctor to assess Mrs Ford's condition and encourage her to sit out of bed for bedmaking, attend to her toilet needs and elimination. Give analgesics when necessary and talk to her.

The second day, continue with the above routine. Help Mrs Ford to walk around her bed. Listen for bowel sounds returning and observe whether naso-gastric aspiration is diminishing. Small amounts of water will be given to her to drink hourly, the naso-gastric tube is spiggoted and aspirated at two hourly intervals. Ask if she has passed flatus. Analgesics may be necessary. Generally her condition should be improving. Observe the amount of fluid and type of fluid aspirated, and note how she tolerates fluids. Report abnormalities.

c   Mrs Ford should be able to cope with normal daily activities before discharge. She should be advised to take small meals with a low carbohydrate content, to chew her meals well, and to rest after meals. She must be told not to swallow large segments of oranges whole. Mrs Ford should be told not to lift heavy objects and to rest. She should contact her general practitioner who may be able to advise that she should have a home help. Before Mrs Ford leaves the hospital an out-patient appointment should be made and she should be given an appointment card with the date and time of the appointment.

4 THE GALL BLADDER

Regional and applied structure and function of the gall bladder.
Fig. 8 shows a diagrammatic representation of the gall bladder and bile ducts. Revise with the aid of your text books, lecture notes and a model. Learn to draw line diagrams and label them correctly. A most useful procedure for describing diseases of the biliary tract.

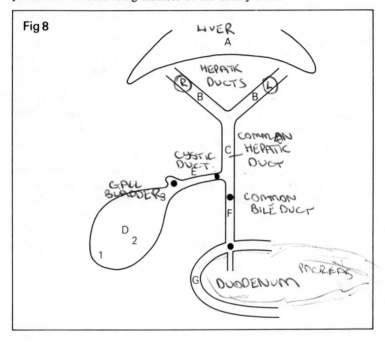

Fig 8

Key.

A the liver
B Rt. and Lt. hepatic ducts
C common hepatic duct
D gallbladder
   1 fundus 2 body 3 neck

E cystic duct
F common bile duct
G duodenum
● Indicates areas most commonly obstructed by gall stones.

Compare and contrast the conditions noted in columns 1, 2 and 3 of Table D on p. 56. Try to work out why these signs and symptoms occur.

The gall bladder is divided into 3 parts, **The fundus,** the body, and the neck. The wall of the gall bladder is composed of smooth muscle lined by mucus membrane. The gall bladder is not essential to life. Its functions are:

a to concentrate bile during its stay in the gall bladder a tenfold increase in concentration occurs.

b to act as a reservoir for bile.

Bile is continuously excreted by the liver, it is stored in the gall bladder as it is only needed during digestion, though emptying of the gall bladder has been observed following sight, smell or taste of food. Nerve fibres from the vagus and sympathetic nerves influence nervous mechanisms; also a hormone called cholecystokinin (which causes the gall bladder to contract) is secreted in response to fatty foods. When the gall bladder contracts, bile is excreted via the cystic duct into the common bile duct, through the sphincter of Oddi into the duodenum. To inhibit contraction and to reduce painful symptoms in gall bladder disease a fat free diet is given.

The main constituents of bile are:

1 water,
2 bile pigments,
3 bile salts,
4 mucus,
5 lecithin,
6 cholesterol,
7 inorganic salts.

The main function of bile is concerned with the digestion and absorption of fat. Stercobilin colours faeces.

Investigations of gall bladder disease

1 Plain X-rays may show a stone in the gall bladder or duct. No preparation is necessary.

2 **Cholecystography Preparation is necessary.**

   a The test is explained to the patient.

   b An iodine preparation, e.g. Telepaque tablets, are given with water the night before the test (iodine is excreted by the liver and concentrated by the gall bladder and is radio opaque, thus the outline of the gall bladder can be seen).

   c The patient is fasted overnight and is taken to the radiography department together with previous notes and X-rays.

   d After the first X-ray is completed a fatty meal is given and more X-rays are taken. A healthy gall bladder will contract in response to a fatty meal, a diseased gall bladder will not contract.

TABLE D   COMMON DISEASES OF THE GALL BLADDER & TOGETHER WITH TYPES OF JAUNDICE

	(1) Acute Cholecystitis	(2) Chronic Cholecystitis
Causes	(1) Usually associated with gall stones. (2) Bacteria i.e. E. Coli Streptococci B. Typhi	Gall stones and a non-functioning gall bladder. Stones may be (a) Cholesterol (b) Mixed (c) Pigment
Sex Incidence Mnemonic	More common in females, fair, fat, forty.	Common in females.
Signs & Symptoms Commonly Experienced	(1) Flatulence, dyspepsia intolerance to fats. (2) Sudden severe pain in rt. hypochondrium radiating through to the back. (3) Nausea (4) Vomiting (5) Raised Temperature	(1) Flatulence, dyspepsia, intolerance of fats (2) Abdominal distension (3) Repeated attacks of pain. Colic in hypochondrium radiating through to back. (4) Jaundice may be a sign (5) Bradycardia + itching if jaundice is present.
Immediate Care & Treatment	(1) Bed rest i.v.i. (2) Naso-gastric aspiration (3) Analgesic (NOT morphia) (4) Antispasmodics (5) Antibiotics (Tetracycline group) (6) Fat free diet.	(1) Bed rest i.v. i. (2) Naso-gastric aspiration (3) Analgesic (NOT morphia) (4) Antispasmodics (5) Antibiotic (6) Fat free diet
Investigation	Plain X-ray H.b. L.F.T. Observation of urine + faeces. Cholecystography.	Plain X-ray H.b. L.F.T. Observation of urine + faeces. i.v. Cholangiogram
Long term treatment	Cholecystectomy	Cholecystectomy and exploration of the common bile duct may be necessary.
Surgical Approach	Abdominal via rt. upper paramedian or Kocker incision.	Abdominal rt. upper paramedian incision.

BILIARY TRACT INVESTIGATIONS & TREATMENTS

(3) Carcinoma of Gall Bladder	Jaundice (4) Pre-hepatic + Hepatic	(5) Post Hepatic
Rare. Gall stones are always present.	(1) Virus (2) Infective hepatitis ⎫ (3) Drugs, Poisons ⎬ hepatic (4) Increased destruction of red blood cells — Pre-hepatic	(1) Gall stones (2) Carcinoma of head of Pancreas (3) Metastases from the stomach
More common in females over 50 years.	Either sex	Either sex
(1) Flatulence, dyspepsia, intolerance of fats (2) Constant insidious pain in the rt. hypochondrium (3) Nausea vomiting malaise (4) Jaundice which deepens looks almost green (5) A mass may be evident	Jaundice which is a yellow discolouration of skin and mucous membrane.	(1) Flatulence, dyspepsia (2) Pain (3) Nausea & vomiting (4) Malaise (5) Weight loss
(1) Bed rest i.v.i. (2) Naso-gastric aspiration (3) Antispasmodics (4) Analgesic	(1) Bed rest (2) Fluids (3) If virus or infective hepatitis isolate and disinfect stools and urine before disposal.	(1) Bed rest i.v.i. (2) Naso-gastric aspiration (3) Analgesics (NOT morphia) (4) Antispasmodics (5) Fat free diet
Plain X-ray H.b. L.F.T. Observation of urine faeces + Jaundice. i.v. Cholangiogram	Liver function tests. Blood picture, L.F.T. blood culture (1) Observation of urine and faeces & Jaundice.	Plain X-ray H.b. Skeletal survey (2) + (3). Liver function test. Blood picture. i.v. Cholangiogram. Observation of jaundice, urine & faeces.
If operable a cholecystectomy may be done and partial hepatectomy. Radiography may be considered or as palliative treatment the gall bladder is joined to the small intestine. Choledochoduodenostomy.	No surgical intervention. The cause is treated if possible.	Treatment of cause. See columns 1, 2 and 3. Work out the treatment for 1, 2 + 3 in this column.
Abdominal rt. upper paramedian incision. Poor prognosis.		

3   **Intravenous Cholangiogram** This investigation entails an injection of an iodine preparation — (see above). The injection outlines the biliary tube and shows if stones or strictures are present.
Positive results from 2 and 3 above.
a Stones will show as filling defects.
b No concentration of dye means the gall bladder is diseased.
N.B. Cholecystography is not done to investigate jaundiced patients as the liver cannot excrete the dye.

4   **Liver function tests.** Tests on venous blood are done to investigate causes of jaundice. Obstructive jaundice caused by obstruction in the common bile duct, usually by stones, will cause back pressure of bile (it cannot get into the duodenum) in the biliary tube which will lead to liver damage. Liver function tests also help differentiate between jaundice due to obstruction of flow of bile, and jaundice due to liver disease.

The most common indication for surgery to the gall bladder is gall stones which cause cholecystitis or blockage of the cystic or common bile ducts.
Please refer to General Pre-operative preparation in chapter 1

Specific preparation for surgery to the gall bladder and bile ducts

If the patient is jaundiced a course of Vitamin K_1 is given intramuscularly, pre-operatively, together with glucose, as carbohydrates protect the liver cells from damage and vitamin K_1 helps prevent bleeding. Routine pre-operative preparations are carried out and a naso-gastric tube is passed. An i.v.i. of Dextrose saline may be started.

During the operation

An operative cholangiogram is done and if stones or strictures are seen the common bile duct is opened the stones are removed and strictures dilated. A T tube is inserted after this procedure into the common bile duct. The gall bladder is removed (cholecystectomy) and a redivac drain is left in the gall bladder region and is brought out through the skin via a stab wound. The drain is attached to a redivac bottle and the abdomen is closed in layers.

If the common bile duct is not opened, only the gall bladder is removed. Some surgeons take out the appendix at this operation, so that the patient may avoid another operation resulting from appendicitis.

Post operative care

Refer to general post-operative care in chapter 1 and care of drains, wounds and naso-gastric tubes in this chapter.

Specific post operative care

When a T tube drain is in place.

1 Inspect the T tube, the patient should not lie on the tube and it should not be obstructed in any way.

2 Measure the amount of bile that drains daily and enter volume on the fluid balance chart.

3 Protect the skin around the stab wound as bile will excoriate the skin.

4 The patient loses electrolytes with bile, therefore his general state must be carefully observed. Blood is taken daily to estimate electrolyte balance.

5 Observation of stools, jaundice and urine are important. Remember that in obstructive jaundice the stools are pale and the urine dark. Jaundice should be receding post-operatively and the stools and urine should return to their normal colour.

6 The T tube is not clamped until the doctor advises.

7 A post-operative cholangiogram is done through the T tube about the 5th to 7th day.

8 After seeing the result of the cholangiogram instruction may be given to clamp the tube at hourly intervals. If the patient does not experience pain the tube is clamped for 12–24 hours. If the temperature of the patient is normal and no pain is experienced after this procedure the T tube is removed when advised by the surgeon. A light diet is started as soon as possible, and full diet should be taken before the patient is discharged home. It is possible that the patient may experience constipation post-operatively and an aperient may be ordered until normal bowel actions are established. The patient may experience dyspepsia post-operatively and be upset by certain food stuffs, they should be told this is not abnormal and that these symptoms will resolve later.

Refer to principles for discharging patients from hospital in this chapter. The after-care of patients who undergo surgery of the gall bladder will be influenced by the reason for surgery, e.g. the patient who has carcinoma may go on to another hospital for radiotherapy.

Practice Questions

Test 3

Test your comprehension of this section of the work by answering the following questions. Do not refer to the answers until you have completed the questions. It may be necessary to re-read the work if you have several answers wrong. Try to draw line diagrams and label them correctly.

1. Which one of the following is an essential clotting factor?
   a Vitamin K_1
   b Progesterone
   c Prothrombin
   d Pitressin

2. Which of the following should not be given to a patient with liver damage?
   a Largactil
   b Pethedine
   c Morphia
   d Pituitrin.

3. Which of the following signs indicates biliary obstruction?
   a Brown constipated stools
   b Clay coloured loose stools
   c Brown coloured loose stools
   d Clay coloured constipated stools.

4. Which of the following signs indicates biliary obstruction?
   a Blood stained urine
   b Yellow frothy urine
   c Pale urine with sediment
   d Green/brown coloured urine.

5. Which of the following is correct? Cholecystectomy and exploration of the common bile duct is the operation of choice for:
   a Obstructive jaundice
   b Hepatic jaundice
   c Pre-hepatic jaundice
   d Haemolytic jaundice

6. Which of the following vitamins cannot be absorbed in the absence of bile?
   a Vitamin A
   b Vitamin B
   c Vitamin D
   d Vitamin K

7. Which of the following hormones causes the gall bladder to contract?
   a Enterogastrone
   b Gastrin
   c Cholecystokinin
   d Pancreozymin
8. Bradycardia is a symptom often seen in
   a Pre-hepatic jaundice
   b Post-hepatic jaundice
   c Haemolytic jaundice
   d Hepatic jaundice.
9. When obstructive jaundice is due to carcinoma of the head of the pancreas which one of the following operations may be performed?
   a Cholecystectomy
   b Cholecystostomy
   c Choledochoduodenostomy
10. What does bradycardia mean?
11. Why is cholecystography sometimes necessary?
12. Why is intravenous cholangiogram necessary?
13. Define the term hepatic jaundice. — jaundice from damaged liver cells
14. Define the term pre-hepatic jaundice. — jaundice from ? break of RB cells down
15. What does insidious in onset mean?
16. Define dyspepsia.
17. Why are antispasmodics used in treating gall bladder colic?
18. What does empyaema mean?
19. What does jaundice mean?
20. Mrs. Kent a 46 year old school teacher is admitted with recurrent cholecystitis. She is in pain, slightly jaundiced and vomiting.
    a Describe the significance of making observations on i) urine, ii) faeces, iii) skin, to a junior nurse.   30%
    b What would be the possible lines of medical treatment given on her admission?   20%
    c Describe the nursing care and management needed by Mrs. Kent during the 48 hours after cholecystectomy and exploration of the common bile duct.   50%

Answers to Test 3

1. c	4. d	7. c
2. a + c	5. a	8. b
3. d	6. d	9. c

10. Bradycardia, a slow pulse rate often found when patients suffer with obstructive jaundice.
11. To investigate the gall bladder for disease and to examine its function.
12. To investigate the gall bladder and biliary tract for disease and to examine its function.
13 Refers to jaundice resulting from damage to liver cells.
14. Refers to jaundice resulting from excessive breakdown of red blood cells.
15. Slow and treacherous in developing.
16. Dyspepsia means indigestion which can be extremely painful.
17. Antispasmodics are given to relieve plain muscle spasm as in biliary colic.
18. Pus in a cavity, a possible complication of cholycystitis.
19. A yellow discoloration of skin and conjunctiva due to excess of bile pigment in the blood.

Model Answer to Question 20

a Explain the normal pathway of bile from the gall bladder to the small intestine, e.g. bile is stored and concentrated in the gall bladder which contracts under the control of (a) nervous factor, e.g. sight, smell and taste of food; (b) humoral factor e.g. fat in the duodenum, cholecystokinin produced. Bile passes via the cystic and common bile duct via the sphincter of Oddi to the small intestine. Bile salts emulsify fat and with pancreatic lipase help absorb fat. Most bile salts are reabsorbed as are some bile pigments. A small amount of bile pigments circulate in the plasma and are excreted in the urine as urobilin. Bacteria in the intestine converts bile pigments to stercobilin which colours faeces brown. If for any reason the flow of bile is obstructed these functions are altered and stools become pale and constipated, urine is brown/green and the skin and conjunctiva are yellow and the skin itches. If changes in stools, urine or skin colour occur they must be reported immediately as an aid to diagnosis.

b 1 Bedrest. 2 Analgesic or Antispasmodic. 3 Nasogastric aspiration. 4 Fluids only or intravenous fluids. 5 Antibiotics. 6 Blood for Hb., group W.C.C., L.F.T. (i.e. S. Bilirubin). 7 Plain X-ray. 8 4 hourly T.P.R. B/P. 9 Observation of stools, urine and skin. 10 Fatfree diet later. Investigations will be done when the acute period is over, i.e. intravenous cholangiogram. Surgery is done when the acute period is resolved.

c   Maintenance of circulation and respiration. Place comfortably in bed, position i.v.i., redivac drain and T tube drain on hangers. Observe wound and vital signs. Report any abnormalities. Give analgesics when necessary and sit the patient up as soon as possible, try to prevent preventable complications, i.e. chest infection, deep vein thrombosis. Observe volume and character of bile and redivac drains and naso-gastric aspiration and record, chart urine passed and test for bile. Reassure Mrs. Kent, give mouth washes and keep her cool and dry. Keep the area round the T tube protected. Let her rest between activities. On the first day help her out of bed for bed-making and observe her vital signs, drains, i.v.i., attend to hygiene, moving and coughing, analgesics may be given. Record all fluid intake and output and balance at the end of the day.

2   On the second day observe for bowel sounds returning. Fluids may be given orally, if Mrs. Kent tolerates fluids the naso-gastric tube may be removed if the doctor advises and possibly the intravenous infusion. She will be much more comfortable then. Help her to walk around the bed, the T tube drainage bag and redivac bottle will have to be carried. Make sure the area around the T tube is dry.

Analgesics may be given if necessary, observe for vital signs, for diminishing jaundice and amount of bile drainage. If drainage from the redivac tube has stopped the drain may be removed.

General hygiene should be attended to. Fluid intake and output should be recorded and observations made of the character of urine passed.

There should be an improvement in ability to move about and breathe deeply after 48 hours.

Any complaints of pain around the site of the wound or the T tube should be investigated.

An elevated temperature may indicate chest or wound infection, or deep vein thrombosis.

Reactionary bleeding can occur, a rise in pulse rate with poor volume, accompanied by pain and sweating may indicate that the patient is bleeding.

Usually the temperature, pulse, respirations and blood pressure are taken and recorded 4 hourly for 4 days post-operatively; significant changes should be reported.

Every attempt should be made to ensure the safety and comfort of the patient so that her recovery may be steady.

5 THE PERITONEUM AND LARGE AND SMALL INTESTINE

For a detailed study refer to models and lecture notes to aid your revision.

The peritoneum is a closed sac within the abdominal cavity. It is the largest serous membrane in the body and is divided into two layers.

a   **The parietal membrane** lines the abdominal wall, it is richly supplied with nerves. If the parietal membrane is irritated pain is experienced in the affected area.

b   **The visceral membrane** covers viscera or organs in the abdominal cavity. Because the two layers are in contact, friction is prevented by secretion of serous fluid. The peritoneum has a complex arrangement and not all of the organs in the abdominal cavity are covered by it, e.g. i the duodenum, kidneys, spleen, pancreas, and pelvic organs are only covered anteriorly;

ii the stomach, liver and intestines are almost enveloped in peritoneum.

Attachments to the posterior abdominal wall influence movement of organs, e.g. the ileum, jejunum, transverse colon and pelvic colon have long attachments and therefore glide smoothly over each other. The ascending colon and duodenum have a short attachment and are fixed. In the male the peritoneal cavity is closed, but the fallopian tubes of the female enter it.

The mesentry
The mesentry describes a double fold of peritoneum which encloses and attaches the small intestine to the posterior abdominal wall. The attachment is short, the small intestine is long, therefore the appearance is known as fan-shaped. The superior mesenteric artery and superior mesenteric vein supply and drain the small intestine via the mesentery. The nerve supply is vagus and sympathetic. The transverse colon is suspended from the transverse **meso-colon**, the meso-colon carries the blood and nerve supply. The pelvic colon is suspended from the **pelvic meso-colon**, blood and nerve supply is mediated via the mesentry.

Lesser omentum
The lesser omentum describes the fold of peritoneum that stretches from the liver to the lesser curve of the stomach.

Greater omentum

The greater omentum is a loose sheet of peritoneum which stores fat and is richly supplied with blood and lymph vessels and lymph nodes. It hangs from the lower border of the stomach like an apron in front of the abdominal organs and reflects back to the posterior abdominal wall. It has a protective function and is sometimes known as the policeman of the abdomen, apart from the presence of lymph nodes, in appendicitis the omentum has the ability to wall off the appendix from the abdominal organs. In the young and old these powers of localising infection and inflammation are reduced e.g. diffuse peritonitis can result from appendicitis.

The functions of peritoneum are:

1   To support and protect organs.
2   To prevent friction.
3   To protect against infection.
4   To store fat.

The acute abdomen

Many abdominal conditions may be classified under this heading. Peritonitis may result from bacterial inflammation, or blood, bile, gastric juice or urine leaking into the peritoneum. Alternatively obstruction of the common bile duct, intestine or ureter may be the cause of pain. On admission the patient's condition is carefully monitored.

1   Changes in vital signs that must be reported are clammyness, pallor, quick shallow respirations and a lowering blood pressure.
2   Vomiting may be due to pain. The patient with appendicitis will vomit once or twice, projectile vomiting in the young child suggests congenital pyloric stenosis. Effortless vomiting of a large volume suggests high intestinal obstruction. Faeculent vomiting is a serious sign of advanced intestinal obstruction. Vomiting occurs once or twice in localized peritonitis, and copious vomiting occurs in paralytic ileus. Haematemesis indicates either injury or erosion of a blood vessel by a peptic ulcer or bleeding from oesophageal varices.
3   Pain should be observed for character and periodicity. In inflammation pain is aching and throbbing in character. The pain of appendicitis becomes more intense. Colic due to obstruction occurs in spasms of increased intensity and pain may be experienced between spasms. Colicky pain is associated with sweating and vomiting and the patient will roll about. The patient with a perforated peptic ulcer will lie still.
4   Bowel function, constipation is a common feature of acute abdominal conditions.

Acute peritonitis

May be due to inflammation, perforation, or interference with blood supply to an intra abdominal organ.

Signs and symptoms

In the early stages of acute peritonitis the patient lies still and complains of continuous intense burning pain over the affected organ and eventually over the abdomen. The pulse and temperature may be slightly raised and vomiting and constipation are present. Later there may be signs of dehydration and toxaemia with a deterioration in vital signs, i.e. high temperature, rapid pulse and respirations. A naso-gastric tube is passed and continuous suction may be necessary and i.v.i. started. Once the diagnosis is established an analgesic is given and usually an intravenous antibiotic. The nurse's role is to reassure the patient, monitor the vital signs carefully and report deterioration and to administer prescribed treatment and make intelligent observations. The patient's progress is assessed by physical improvement, improved pulse rate and blood pressure and hydration. The patient is prepared for theatre. **See General Principles of pre-operative care in chapter 1.** A mid-line or paramedian laparotomy incision is made so that any eventuality can be dealt with.

See General Principles of Post-operative Care in chapter 1.

Specific post-operative care

1 Observation of vital signs. Improvement is shown by a rise in blood pressure and fall in pulse rate and temperature.
2 Gastric aspiration. Improvement is shown by a marked decrease in the volume and a return to normal bile aspirations from offensive aspirations.
3 The abdomen. Improvement is shown when the abdomen becomes soft and bowel sounds are heard.

Accurate fluid balance charts must be kept and urine specific gravity should be measured.

Anxiety and pain should be relieved by analgesics and the patient should rest easily. Regular breathing exercises and coughing should be encouraged together with leg movements.

The complications of peritonitis are **a** acute intestinal obstruction from adhesions, **b** paralytic ileus, **c** pelvic or subphrenic abscesses.

TABLE E

Intestinal Obstruction may be →

	Adynamic	Dynamic
Causes	Peritonitis · Infective · Post-operative · Reflex · Uraemia	**Acute** **Acute or Chronic** 1) In the lumen of the intestine — gall stones, Crohn's disease, food bolus } most common 2) In the wall 3) Outside the wall — Hernia, Adhesions } most common, Volvulus, Intussusception *Acute or Chronic* (1) Constipation (2) Distension (3) Pain (4) Vomiting
Signs & Symptoms	(1) Rise in temperature (2) Rise in pulse rate (3) Abdominal pain (4) Vomiting (5) Rigid, tender abdomen	*Acute* (1) Pain (2) Vomiting (3) Distension (4) Constipation
Immediate Treatment	(1) N.G. aspiration (3) Sedation (2) i.v.i. (4) Antibiotics	(1) N.G. Aspiration (2) i.v.i. (3) Sedation when cause is established.
Investigation	Plain X-ray Blood for blood picture. If bacteriaemia blood for culture and sensitivity.	Plain X-ray for fluid levels Blood for blood count Hb Group electrolytes
Treatment	Of the primary cause.	Relieve the obstruction surgically Treat primary cause
	Strangulation of the bowel occurs when it is trapped by (a) A band (b) A hernia (c) Intussusception (d) Volvulus in such a way that the blood supply is interfered with. This is a very dangerous condition and early treatment is necessary.	

Acute appendicitis

Appendicitis is a common surgical emergency in the 10-30 year old age group.

Classically the features are:

1   Pain that originates around the umbilicus and localises in the right iliac fossa.
2   Anorexia and nausea, there may be a characteristic smell on the breath.
3   One or two episodes of vomiting.
4   A normal or slight rise in temperature, and a normal or slight rise in pulse rate.
5   There is guarding and tenderness over the right iliac fossa.

On admission the patient is put to bed and made as comfortable as possible, a history of his normal physical abilities are taken. The doctor examines the patient and a rectal examination is mandatory. Urine passed is recorded and tested and the vital signs are taken and recorded hourly. A mouthwash is given and the patient is reassured. Blood is taken for grouping Hb and full cell count.

Indications for surgery are fever, leucocytosis and guarding. Nowadays, treatment is usually surgical.

Perforated appendix

This must be treated immediately as delay results in more extensive peritonitis.

Appendix abscess

It is usual to wait for the abscess to subside. The appendix is removed in about three months when all the inflammation has subsided.

See General Principles of Pre-operative and Post-operative care in chapter 1. Refer to previous notes.

Complications following appendicectomy are:

1   Pelvic abscess
2   Paralytic ileus
3   Intestinal obstruction.

Differential diagnoses to appendicitis are **a** twisted or ruptured ovarian cyst, **b** Crohn's disease, **c** acute non-specific mesenteric adenitis, most common in children, **d** pyelitis, **e** Meckel's diverticulum.

The structure and function of the small and large intestine.

Revise thoroughly with the aid of textbooks, lecture notes and models. Learn to draw line diagrams and label them correctly.

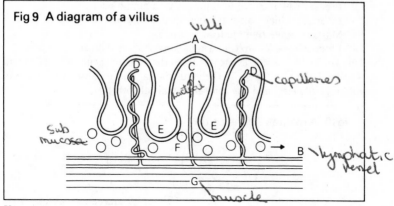

Fig 9 A diagram of a villus

Key
A Villi
B Lymphatic vessel
C Central lacteal
D Capillaries
E Intestinal gland
F Submucosa
G Muscle

The small intestine stretches from the pyloric sphincter (which prevents backflow of intestinal juices into the stomach) to the ileocaecal valve (which prevents backflow from the colon into the ileum). The duodenum is the first part, about 10″ long leading from the stomach to the jejunum. Here chyme is mixed with bile and pancreatic juices. The jejunum and ileum, 8ft and 12ft long respectively, continue on from the duodenum.

The structure of the small intestine

As with the stomach the small intestine has four coats.
1. Peritoneum, 2. muscle, 3. sub-mucous, 4. mucous. The arrangement differs from that of the stomach as the muscle coat has only two layers.
1. longitudinal, 2. circular.
The mucous membrane is arranged in circular folds which do not flatten out when the intestine distends. These folds increase the surface area of the small intestine so that secretion and absorption can take place. In the mucous membrane are large numbers of glands secreting intestinal juice — succus entericus an alkaline fluid containing:

1   Erepsin which converts peptones into amino acids.
2   Invertase which converts cane sugar into glucose.
3   Maltase converting maltose to glucose.
4   Enterokinase an enzyme which converts trypsinogen to trypsin.

Tiny finger-like processes project from the mucous membrane called villi — (see diagram in Fig 9). In the villus the capilliaries absorb glucose and amino acids, etc., and the central lacteals absorb fats.

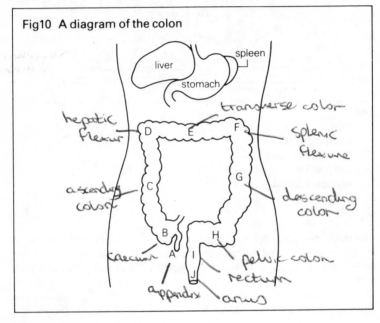

Fig10   A diagram of the colon

Key

A   Appendix
B   Caecum
C   Ascending colon
D   Hepatic flexure
E   Transverse colon
F   Splenic colon
G   Descending colon
H   Pelvic colon
I   Rectum
J   Anus

There are numerous lymph nodes dotted about, the most important lymph nodes are Peyer's patches situated toward the distal portion. These are inflamed in typhoid fever. Movements of the intestine are peristaltic, segmenting and pendular. Blood supply and venous drainage are via mesenteric arteries and veins.

Steatorrhoea is a symptom of malabsorption in the small intestine which may arise **a from inadequate digestion,** i pancreatic insufficiency, ii inactivation of pancreatic enzymes, iii after polya-gastrectomy, etc; **b mucosal cell disorders**, e.g. i coeliac disease, ii Whipple's disease, iii intestinal ischaemia, iv Crohn's disease. The patient complains of frequent passage of semi-formed stools or liquid stools, stools are greasy, there is weight loss, anorexia, anaemia is common and vitamins are not absorbed with resultant deficiency diseases if not corrected. Treatment is of cause, if possible.

The large intestine or colon

The colon starts at the caecum in the right iliac fossa and ends at the anal canal. It has six parts:
1   the caecum and appendix.
2   the ascending colon.
3   the transverse colon.
4   the descending colon.
5   the pelvic colon.
6   the rectum and anal canal (see Fig. 10).

Structure of the large intestine

Similarly structured to the other parts of the tract, i.e. 1. peritoneum, 2. muscular, 3. sub-mucous and 4. mucous. The muscle layer differs from that of the stomach and small intestine as the longitudinal muscle fibres are arranged in three separate bands. The bands are shorter in length than the colon and give a sacculated appearance. When the longitudinal fibres reach the rectum they spread out over the whole area. The mucous membrane does not contain villi, is not thrown into folds. It is lined by columnar epithelium with many goblet cells secreting mucus.

Blood supply

The upper portion of the colon is supplied by the superior mesenteric artery, the lower portion including the rectum is supplied by the inferior mesenteric artery. Venous drainage is by the superior and inferior mesenteric veins.

Nerve supply
This is mediated by vagus and sympathetic nerves.

Function of the colon

1   To secrete mucus to lubricate faeces.
2   Nothing of nutritional value is prepared in the colon but products such as amino acids which have not been absorbed in the small intestine undergo bacterial decomposition, Vit. B and K are synthesised.
3   Large quantities of water are absorbed.
4   It converts the fluid contents of the small intestine into faeces.

As food is taken into the stomach the ileo-caecal valve relaxes and the contents of the ileum are passed into the caecum by peristaltic action. This is called the gastro-colic reflex. There is general peristaltic action throughout the colon. The contents of the colon enter the rectum which distends, nerve endings are stimulated and impulses pass to the spinal cord and on to the brain and there is a conscious desire to empty the bowel. Failure to respond to this process usually results in constipation. Change in bowel habit is an important symptom of disease in the bowel, and can also be significant of disease in the pancreas, thyroid, etc.

Using Table F, compare and contrast Crohn's disease with ulcerative colitis. Compare and contrast carcinoma of the colon with diverticulitis.

Preparation of patients for surgery to the intestine
See General Principles of pre-operative care in chapter 1
specific preparation for elective surgery
For operations on the intestine it is necessary:

1   To sterilise the bowel by oral administration of e.g. sulphonamides or antibiotics. The surgeon prescribes his preference for medication, as they do not all agree about the use of certain drugs.
2   To wash out the bowel twice daily starting three days pre-operatively. The patient is given a nutritious diet when the bowel preparation begins.

If there is severe haemorrhage or perforation of the intestine this preparation will not be carried out. Treatment of disease in the small and large intestine sometimes necessitates establishing a temporary or permanent opening in the bowel so that intestinal contents are discharged onto the abdominal wall. The opening is called a stoma. An ileostomy means that the end of the terminal ileum is brought out onto the right side of the abdominal wall. A colostomy is the opening of the colon onto the abdominal wall, usually on the left side of the abdominal wall.

When ileostomy or colostomy of a permanent type is advised pre-operatively by the surgeon, time must be given to explain carefully the intended procedure and to reassure the patient. The patient must be helped to come to terms with the idea. Most patients are upset, some are extremely distressed, and others will not accept that this is happening to them. Common fears are that after the operation they will not be acceptable in society, or by their marriage partner, or of ability to cope post-operatively. It is important to help the patient talk about his fears. When he is accustomed to the idea it may be advisable to request a visit from an established ileostomist or colostomist, (the Ileostomy Association provide this service freely) and if possible a person of the patient's own age group. It can make a difference to the way the patient accepts the procedure. There is a wealth of literature available nowadays for information of ostomists, mostly available in bookshops. When the patient is ready to discuss the equipment the range available should be discussed with him. The disposable equipment available is fairly easy to handle and dispose of and can't be seen under clothing. Usually the surgeon will decide on the site of the stoma pre-operatively and it may be necessary for the skin to be marked pre-operatively.

See General Principles of post-operative care in chapter 1

Specific care after ileostomy
(Usually an ileostomy is a permanent procedure, very occasionally a temporary ileostomy is performed.)

Fluid balance may be a problem post-operatively as so much fluid is lost from the ileum in the immediate post-operative period. The volume lost in 24 hours is replaced in 24 hours by the intravenous route. Blood for haemaglobin and electrolytes is taken daily and abnormalities must be corrected.

An ileostomy bag will be fitted by the surgeon in the theatre and every attempt must be made to keep the appliance in position for as long as possible. Ileostomy bags are drainable and need not be removed unless they come off. The bag will need to be drained frequently in the immediate post-operative period to prevent leakage. If intestinal juice comes into contact with the patient's skin it will excoriate the skin and the patient will suffer unnecessary discomfort. Gas in the bag may cause the

TABLE F   COMMON DISEASES OF THE SMALL & LARGE

	(1) Crohn's disease	(2) Ulcerative Colitis
Cause	Unknown. Can occur anywhere in the alimentary tract. Common in small and large intestine, a disease of remissions and exacerbations.	Unknown. Both colon and rectum may be involved. A disease of remissions and exacerbations.
Sex Incidence	All age groups. Either sex.	All age groups. More common in females.
Signs and Symptoms Problems Experienced	(1) Pain colicky in nature. (2) Diarrhoea, bleeding unusual. (3) Fever & Anorexia. (4) Weight loss. (5) Anaemia. (6) Skin lesions. (7) Anal lesions. Recurrent obstructions are common.	(1) Diarrhoea mucous and blood stained. (2) Colicky pain. (3) Fever & Anorexia. (4) Weight loss. (5) Anaemia. (6) Rarely Anal lesions. Malignant disease may occur.
Investigations	Plain X-ray. Rectal examination. Sigmoidoscopy. Barium Enema, Barium meal and biopsy. Blood picture. Stools for occult blood fats E.S.R.	Plain X-ray. Rectal examination. Sigmoidoscopy and biopsy. Barium Enema. Blood picture. E.S.R.
Treatment	Initially medical. Drugs are given to produce remission. Steroids, Salazopyrin Folic. vit. C vit. D. Iron to correct deficiency. Prednisone enemas.	Initially medical. Drugs are given to bring about remission. Steroids salazopyrin. Iron. Prednisone enemas to reduce inflammation locally.
	Patients who are to undergo surgery to the large bowel should have antibiotics and bowel washouts	
Surgical Treatment Depends on site of lesion	(1) A bypass operation may be done. (2) Total colectomy with ileostomy is more usual.	(1) Colectomy and Ileostomy (2) Complete excision of colon and rectum and ileostomy

INTESTINE INVESTIGATIONS & TREATMENT

(3) Carcinoma	(4) Diverticulitis	(5) Haemorrhoids
Adenocarcinoma	Thought to be associated with low fibre diet. There is incoordination between rectum and bowel.	Varicose vein, not known may be an hereditary factor. Usually results from pressure, i.e. pregnancy or constipation.
Older age group. Slightly more common in females.	Both sexes over forty years.	Both sexes over 30 years.
Depends on site of lesion. Alteration of bowel habit. (1) Rectal lesion. Sensation of incomplete defaecation. Fresh blood in stools. (2) In descending colon alternating diarrhoea and constipation. (3) Pain may be related to meals in lesions of the ascending colon. Pain may not be felt until late in Ca. of rectum. (4) Weight loss anaemia.	(1) Pain in left iliac fossa. (2) Alternating diarrhoea and constipation. (3) Fever.	(1) Rectal bleeding. (2) Pain. (3) Constipation. (4) Prolapse of piles.
Plain X-ray. Blood picture. Rectal examination. Sigmoidoscopy and biopsy. Barium enema.	Plain X-ray. Blood picture. Rectal examination. Sigmoidoscopy. Barium enema.	Rectal examination. Sigmoidoscopy.
Surgical and radiotherapy.	Initially medical aperients are given and a high fibre diet.	Initially observation. Aperients are given. Local injection of piles.
treatment to sterilise the bowel, i.e. sulphanamides and		
Carcinoma in the rectum — Removal of rectum, with colostomy. Hemi-colectomy of the affected area.	(1) Removal of diseased part of bowel if symptoms are distressing or haemorrhage occurs. (2) If perforation occurs a loop colostomy is done and resection later.	Haemorrhoidectomy.

bag to leak or lift off the skin surface, a small pin prick at the top end of the bag may help solve the problem. Most gastro-enterology departments have the services of a stoma therapist who will be able to spend time with the patient, and advise on fitting, suitable equipment and instruct the patient in applying the equipment. As soon as the patient is able he should be encouraged to look at the ileostomy and to change the appliance so that confidence is gained.

1   The skin around the ileostomy must be kept dry. A sore wet skin is uncomfortable and can be painful and lead to difficulties in sticking on the appliances, resulting in psychological problems. There are several products available for dealing with the problems of adhesion.
2   The stoma should be measured for prolapse or changes in colour and the correct sized ring used. Skin should not be visible inside the ring.
3   **Remember that the efficiency with which the ileostomy is handled in the first few post-operative days can influence the patient's recovery rate and development of confidence.**
4   Before the patient is discharged he/she must be:
   a Fitted with the equipment most suitable for his needs
   b Able to change the appliances
   c Able to cope with problems of leakage
   d Instructed in the diet most suitable to prevent leaking. Isogel taken before meals can help thicken the contents of the ileum.
   e Able to order equipment from a local chemist.
   f Instructed about his medication.
5   The patient should be encouraged to join the Ileostomy Association so that he does not feel isolated with his problem.
6   An appointment must be made for the out-patient's department.

Specific care after colostomy
(colostomy may be temporary or permanent)

The transverse or descending colon are the sites commonly chosen for colostomy.

The temporary loop colostomy will be opened about 3/4 days post-operatively in the ward using diathermy, when the peritoneum has healed so that faeces will not contaminate the abdominal cavity. The problems encountered in the post-operative period are similar to that of the ileostomy patient, but the fluid content of the transverse and descending colon is rather thicker than that of the ileum. Therefore loss of fluid is not so much of a problem.

Some surgeons do not apply a colostomy bag in the operating theatre and the colostomy is surrounded by dressings which must be changed when soiled. The abdominal wound must be sealed in this case to prevent faecal contamination. The same care as for the ileostomy patient must be given to the colostomist who will experience similar psychological problems.

Irrigations of colostomy are sometimes necessary. In some instances the bowel action becomes so controlled the patient does not have to wear a bag. The type of colostomy bag used is not drainable.

There is less likelihood of complications arising from a colostomy than an ileostomy. Careful observations have to be made of the stoma in both cases for alteration in colour, or prolapse. If the rectum has been removed the patient will have three wounds to cope with:

1 an abdominal wound
2 a perineal wound
3 colostomy.

The abdominal wound and perineal wound will be drained and drainage must be assessed. Probably the perineal wound will need extra packing applied in the first 24 hours post-operatively and a T binder helps secure these dressings tightly in place. The problems in the post-operative period are:

a position for most comfort
b re-packing and irrigation of the perineal wound
c the perineal wound may not heal quickly.

Patients having surgery in the pelvis will have a catheter inserted pre-operatively and this will remain *in situ* for several days post-operatively. There may be incontinence when the catheter is removed.

Refer to section on ileostomy for discharge procedure.

Practice Questions

Test 4

Test your comprehension of this section of the work by answering the following questions. Complete the test, then check your answers.

1. What is the function of the peritoneum?
2. What types of vomiting suggest
   a Pyloric stenosis
   b High intestinal obstruction
   c Advanced intestinal obstruction?
3. Describe the pain characteristics of
   a Inflammation
   b Colic
   c Perforated peptic ulcer.
4. List the early signs of acute peritonitis.
5. List the causes of adynamic intestinal obstruction.
6. List the causes of dynamic intestinal obstruction.
7. List the signs and symptoms of acute intestinal obstruction.
8. List the signs and symptoms of acute or chronic intestinal obstruction.
9. List the signs and symptoms of acute appendicitis.
10. List the investigations necessary in diagnosis of acute appendicitis.
11. Name the parts of the small intestine.
12. How does the structure of the small intestine differ from that of the stomach?
13. What is the function of the small intestine?
14. How does the structure of the large intestine differ from the structure of the small intestine?
15. What is the function of the large intestine?
16. What is malabsorption a sign of?
17. What is steatorrhoea a symptom of?
18. What does steatorrhoea mean?
19. State the type of bowel action most common in acute intestinal obstruction.
20. Describe the type of bowel action experienced with diverticulitis.
21. What may fresh blood in the stools indicate?
22. What drugs are used to treat patients with Crohn's disease?
23. What may alternating diarrhoea and constipation indicate?
24. List the common signs and symptoms of Crohn's disease.
25. What investigations are necessary to diagnose conditions of the large intestine?

26. What complications may occur in Crohn's disease?
27. State the treatment of haemorrhoids.
28. State the complications of ulcerative colitis.
29. Describe the bowel action indicative of Crohn's disease.
30. Describe the bowel action indicative of ulcerative colitis.
31. What drugs are used to treat patients with ulcerative colitis?
32. State the types of operations performed for ulcerative colitis.
33. State the operations performed for Crohn's disease.
34. State the conservative treatment for diverticulitis.
35. State the type of operations performed for carcinoma of the rectum.
36. What does ileostomy mean?
37. What does colostomy mean?
38. State the specific preoperative preparation necessary for bowel surgery.
39. John aged 18 years is admitted with obstruction of the intestine from Crohn's disease.
    a What immediate treatment would John be given, and what would signify an improvement in his condition?
    b What are the signs, symptoms and complications of Crohn's disease?
    c What advice would you give to John who has a newly performed ileostomy?

Answers to Test 4

1. To support and protect organs in the abdominal cavity. To protect against infection. To prevent friction and to store fat.
2. a Projectile or forcibly projected vomit.
   b Copious effortless vomit.
   c Faeculent vomit.
3. a Aching and throbbing.
   b Occurs in spasms causing patient to roll around.
   c Increases in intensity, is burning, the patient does not move as movement increases the pain.
4. Continuous, intense, burning pain over the affected organ. Slight rise in pulse and temperature, vomiting and constipation present.
5. i Infection ii Post-operative iii Uraemia iv Reflex, i.e. injuries to the spine or from being encased in paster spica.
6. i In the lumen, food or gall stones.
   ii In the wall, Crohn's disease.
   iii Outside the wall, hernia, adhesions, volvulus intussusception.

7. Pain, vomiting, distension, constipation.
8. Constipation, distension, pain, vomiting.
9. Pain and guarding in the right iliac fossa, anorexia and nausea with characteristic smell on the breath. A slight rise in temperature and pulse rate.
10. A rectal examination. Blood. Hb full blood count. In acute appendicitis there is leucocytosis.
11. Duodenum. Jejunum. Ileum.
12. The muscle coat has two layers, longitudinal and circular.
    The mucous coat has circular folds (valulae conniventes), which do not flatten when the gut distends. The muscle coat of the stomach has three layers. The mucous membrane or rougae flattens when the stomach distends.
13. Moves contents forward by peristaltic, segmental and pendular movements, secretes intestinal juice, completes digestion, protects against infection.
14. The muscle layer has longitudinal bands of muscle fibres (taema coli) which give a puckered appearance to the colon as they are slightly shorter in length than the colon.
15. Absorption of water and some glucose and mineral salts. Synthesis of vitamins B and K. Excretion of iron bismuth.
    Defaecation.
16. Disease in the small intestine.
17. Indicates malabsorption of fats and other essential nutrients.
18. The passage of liquid fat in the stools which are offensive, grey or yellow.
19. Constipation is the most common feature.
20. Alternating diarrhoea and constipation.
21. Bleeding haemorrhoids or rectal carcinoma.
22. Salazopyrin and Steroids. Prednisone enemas may be given to control local inflammation.
23. Diverticulitis or carcinoma in the colon.
24. Colicky pain, diarrhoea, anorexia, weight loss, anaemia, anal fissure, skin lesions.
25. General history, account of bowel habit change, general examination, rectal examination, Sigmoidoscopy, biopsy, barium enema, barium meal and follow through.
26. Malabsorption of vitamins and iron and other essential nutrients, low plasma protein, rectal fissures, obstruction — skip lesions (see Kantor's String Sign). It is a disease of recurrence and remissions.

27. Conservative. Aperients, high fibre diet, local injection.
    Surgical haemorrhoidectomy.
28. Anaemia, weight loss, obstruction, perforation of gut.
    Carcinoma.
29. Frequent stools, in an acute state may be × 20 a day.
    Watery, offensive, not usually blood stained but can be.
30. Frequent stools in an acute state. Watery with mucus and blood,
    perhaps × 20 a day.
31. Salazopyrin. Steroids. Prednisone enemas are given to reduce local
    inflammation.
32. Colectomy and ileostomy. Complete excision of colon and rectum
    with ileostomy. Ileo rectal anastomosis may be done.
33.   i Where an obstruction occurs the gut may be resected, a
        colostomy may be done if the descending colon is involved.
     ii The obstruction may be bypassed internally.
    iii Colectomy with ileostomy most common line of treatment, the
        rectal stump is usually left intact.
34. Aperients and high fibre diet, weight reduction if necessary.
35. Abdominal perineal resection, commonly. Depending on situ an
    anterior resection or Lloyd Davies may be done.
36. Opening into the ileum.
37. Opening into the colon.
38. Bowel washouts and drugs to sterilise the bowel.

Model answer to question 39

a John would be put into bed and made as comfortable as possible.
Vital signs would be taken and recorded and general observations of
his condition made. He may be de-hydrated and his abdomen may
be distended. If the obstruction is in the small intestine he probably
will be vomiting quite copiously.

Medical treatment
A naso-gastric tube is passed, continuous suction may be applied, an
intravenous infusion is commenced and steroids given to try to
reduce inflammation. John's progress would be carefully
monitored. Signs of improvement in the condition would be
reducing amounts of fluid being aspirated, bowel sounds would be
heard and the abdomen would be less distended.

b Diarrhoea, colicky pain, fever, anaemia, loss of weight, anorexia,
anal fissures, skip lesions in the bowel, i.e. diseased sections of gut

are separated by healthy sections of gut. Acute obstruction. Acute or chronic obstruction.

c   The ileostomy.

i   To prevent the skin becoming sore.

ii   To be certain that the ring is the right size for the stoma.

iii   To change the appliance only when necessary (there is no problem with odour with the plastic appliances).

iv   To avoid meals late at night (there may be a problem with leakage at night).

v   To avoid foods that cause diarrhoea.

vi   To join the Ileostomy Society, where up to date information about Crohn's disease and appliances would be available.

vii   Psychologically encourage him to meet his friends and indulge in his usual activities.

viii   To contact the hospital immediately if he is worried about his ileostomy or his general condition.

ix   To take his medication regularly and as prescribed.

6 THE SPLEEN

The objectives of this section are to state:
1 The structure and function of the spleen
2 The reasons for splenectomy
3 The ways in which rupture of the spleen is dealt with.

Structure of the spleen

The spleen is a small organ slightly ovoid in shape composed of lymphoid tissue and blood vessels. It is covered anteriorly by peritoneum. Surrounding the gland is a fibro-elastic capsule and fibrous tissue forms trabeculae within it. The spleen is situated in the left upper abdominal cavity. It is not essential to life and splenectomy does not leave ill-effects.

The function of the spleen
a To form lymphocytes important in body defence.
b To destroy worn out red blood cells.

Splenectomy is indicated when
a The spleen is ruptured.
b During gastrectomy if metastases are present.
c During pancreatectomy — the splenic vessels are destroyed.
d Haemolytic disease is present.
e Idiopathic thrombocytopenia is present.

Rupture of the spleen

This is commonly caused by road traffic accidents i.e. direct injury, or falling from a height, indirect injury.

Signs and symptoms are:
1 Pain which may radiate to the top of the shoulder worsening on deep breathing (sub-diaphragmatic irritation).
2 There is pallor and sweating.
3 There is tachycardia and loss of pulse volume.
4 There may be low systolic blood pressure.

Investigations necessary will be plain X-ray. Blood is taken for Hb P.C.V. Blood group.

A naso-gastric tube is passed to empty and deflate the stomach. If it is thought that the patient has a ruptured spleen on the evidence presented, an emergency splenectomy is performed.

Refer to basic principles of pre-operative care in chapter 1
Surgical approach is via left upper paramedian or left subcostal incision. A redivac drainage tube will be put in place post-operatively. A blood transfusion will be necessary to restore blood volume.

See basic principles of post-operative care in chapter 1
The naso-gastric tube must be aspirated regularly as haematemesis may result from gastric irritation. Breathing exercises must be commenced as soon as possible as atelectasis with pleural effusion may complicate recovery. Persistent hiccough sometimes occurs as a result of irritation of the phrenic nerve. **Paralytic ileus, a serious complication,** should be watched for.

Practice Questions

Test 5

Test your comprehension of this section of the work by answering the following questions. Answer all of the questions in writing then check the answers. If you have several answers wrong, re-read the work.

1. What does haematemesis mean?
2. What does atelectasis mean?
3. What does the term **paralytic ileus** describe?
4. What does the term **splenectomy** mean?
5. Define metastases
6. What does P.C.V. mean?
7. What does idiopathic mean?
8. Why are lymphocytes important?
9. What does thrombocytopaenia mean?
10. Peter aged 12 years falls from a tree. He is admitted with a suspected rupture of the spleen.
    - **a** explain the importance of observations and investigations which may be carried out in the casualty unit.   45%
    - **b** describe his nursing care and management following splenectomy.   55%

Answers to Test 5

1. Haematemesis means vomiting blood from the stomach.
2. Term used to describe collapse of part of the lung.
3. A non-functioning ileum caused by paralysis of the muscle. It may be due to handling of the gut during surgery, or peritonitis.
4. Removal of the spleen.
5. Spread of malignant cells from the primary growth.
6. Packed cell volume, gives a more accurate estimation of blood loss after a sudden haemorrhage than the haemoglobin level.
7. Idiopathic means there is no established cause of disease.
8. Lymphocytes are important in the body defence mechanisms (immunity).
9. Deficiency in numbers of platelets in circulation.

Model Answer to Question 10

a on admission to the casualty unit Peter is made as comfortable as possible and he is assessed by the casualty officer. A history should be taken from his parents.

Investigations. To establish a firm diagnosis.

i   Plain X-ray of abdomen and chest to examine spleen and ribs.
ii Blood is taken for group and cross matching and P.C.V. packed cell volume gives a better guide of blood lost from the circulation in accidental injury than haemoglobin level.

Observations will include:
1. **vital signs taken frequently**
   a pallor
   b tachycardia with poor volume
   c increased respiratory rate with pain and lowering blood pressure are all signs of internal bleeding. If these signs occur they must be reported immediately.

2.a observation of pain: a typical sign of a ruptured spleen is pain that radiates to the tip of the shoulder, due to irritation under the diaphragm from blood.
If the signs of ruptured spleen are positive, consent for operation will be obtained from his parents and an emergency splenectomy will be performed.

b On return to the ward Peter will be placed gently into bed and one pillow is put under his head. Reassure him and check the outer-dressing for bleeding and inspect the drainage, secure the redivac bottle beside the bed. Observe the infusion or transfusion and the site of injection, check the fingers and bandages. Aspirate the naso-gastric tube and record fluid balance, chart urine passed and test urine. Vital signs must be checked frequently and significant changes should be reported. Sit Peter up as soon as possible and start deep breathing exercises as rigorously as he can, as collapse of part of the lung is a possible complication. Any sign of difficulty in breathing or cyanosis must be reported.
Observation of the naso-gastric aspiration is important. Blood stained aspirate may indicate haematemesis from gastric aspiration. Increased gastric aspirations with abdominal rigidity may indicate paralytic ileus has occurred.
Reassure Peter. Spend time with him. Keep him cool with clean linen. Attend to skin hygiene and give oral toilet. Analgesics should be given as ordered. Usually children are more resilient than adults and they start to move about quite freely. Parents should be encouraged to visit freely. If all goes well in about 48 hours and when the doctor advises and when fluid is tolerated and bowel

sounds return, the naso-gastric tube and i.v.i. are removed. The redivac drain is removed when drainage stops. Peter should be helped to walk about and mix with other children as soon as possible. His haemoglobin level is checked and abdominal sutures removed about the 8th or 9th day according to the state of his wound.

If Peter makes an uneventful recovery he should be discharged home about the 10th day. His parents are given a full explanation and advice with regard to exercise, and an out-patient appointment is made.

7 THE RENAL TRACT

The objectives of this section are to state:
1 The regional and applied anatomy of the renal tract
2 Conditions commonly associated with the kidney, ureter, urethra and prostate gland.
3 The management and treatment of patients undergoing surgery of the renal tract.
For a detailed study of A. and P. of renal tract study your lecture notes and textbooks.

The cells of the body need to have a constant normal environment if they are to function properly.
The kidneys form **urine** by a process which can be divided into three phases:
a simple glomerular filtration which is non-selective i.e. regardless of the body's requirements, all those substances in the blood which are of a small molecular size are filtered into the kidney tubules.
b selective tubular reabsorption, which varies according to the needs of the body at any given time.
c tubular secretion, substances in the blood which were not filtered out in the glomerulus can be secreted out into the convoluted tubules by active transport. Surplus acids and alkalis and some drugs are passed out from the blood by this means.
The formation of urine, therefore, performs three functions that are

Essential to health:
 i it helps maintain a water balance in the body
 ii it helps maintain an electrolyte balance in the plasma
iii it helps maintain the pH of the blood at 7.4.

The kidneys and ureters
There are two kidneys each situated behind the peritoneum, one on each side of the vertebral column. The right kidney is usually slightly lower than the left due to the position of the liver.
They are bean-shaped organs, embedded in fat. The kidney and renal fat are enclosed in the renal fascia, a sheath of fibro-elastic tissue.
The right and left supra-renal or adrenal glands lie on the upper border of each kidney. The kidneys are described as having an outer cortex and an

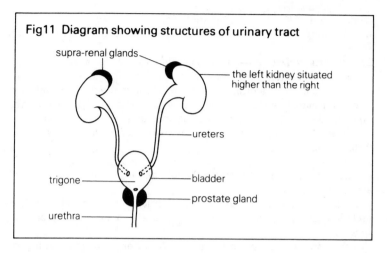

Fig11 Diagram showing structures of urinary tract

supra-renal glands

the left kidney situated higher than the right

ureters

trigone

bladder

prostate gland

urethra

inner medulla and each of them contains about a million **nephrons**. Urine which is formed within the nephrons is passed into collecting ducts and on to the ureters for storage in the urinary bladder until it is excreted.

The kidneys and ureters can be damaged by:
1 **trauma** — a kidney can be ruptured as a result of a direct blow.
2 **infection** — commonly by ascending infection of the urinary tract.
   pyelitis — inflammation of the renal pelvis
   hydronephrosis — dilatation of the renal pelvis due to obstruction to the outflow of urine which predisposes to infection.
   hydroureter — dilatation of the ureter above an obstruction.
3 **stone formation** — within the kidney tubules may cause obstruction inside the kidney or ureters.
4 **tumour formation**
Because of their close proximity to the lower part of the uterus and upper vagina, the ureters may be damaged during operations on these organs. Observation of urinary output is therefore vitally important following such operations.
Operations on the kidneys and ureters include:
nephrectomy — complete removal of the kidney
partial nephrectomy — removal of part of the kidney
nephro-ureterectomy — removal of kidney and ureter
nephrostomy — drainage of the kidney

nephrolithotomy — removal of stone from the kidney
ureterostomy — opening of the ureter via abdominal incision to remove a stone
ureteric catheterization — via a cystoscopy to dislodge a stone
ureteric transplantation — in severe bladder conditions, it might be necessary to perform a urinary diversion. The ureters would be implanted into an isolated portion of the ileum which is brought out to the abdominal wall. The urine is then collected into an ileostomy bag.

There are three important symptoms associated with diseases of the urinary tract.

a Pain
Kidney pain is felt most often in the loin and is usually a constant dull ache.

Ureteric pain is most often due to obstruction and attempts by the ureteric walls to dislodge the obstruction. It is a colicky pain, severe and spasmodic.

Bladder pain ranges from a feeling of discomfort through to strangury which is the extremely painful passage of small amounts of blood stained urine.

Urethral pain is usually described as scalding on micturition.

Prostatic pain is commonly felt in the rectum or perineum.

b Frequency
The patient complains of passing small amounts of urine often.

c Haematuria
The passage of blood in the urine may be painless or painful, the urine may be slightly or heavily bloodstained.

Specific investigations associated with surgery of the kidneys and ureters
These would be preceded by a careful taking of the patient's history and full physical examination.

Urine Tests
 i Routine ward urine test for abnormal constituents.
 ii Specimens to the laboratory for analysis, culture and sensitivity
 iii 24 hour collections for creatinine clearance test (this is a measurement of the glomerular filtration rate — normal clearance is between 80–120 mls/min.)
 iv Specific gravity estimation (this tests the ability of the kidney to concentrate and dilute urine.)
 v Estimation of the patient's total intake and output of fluids over 24 hours. (Strict fluid balance recordings also gives the frequency with which urine is passed and the volume of urine passed each voiding.

Blood tests
The full range of routine tests including regular urea and electrolyte estimation.

Radiological tests
Straight abdominal X-rays
Intravenous pyelography
Infusion pyelogram
Renal arteriography and tomography
Cystography and retrograde pyelography

Endoscopy
Cystoscopy
Cystoscopy combined with retrograde pyelography/ureteric catheterization

Injury to the kidney

The extent of the kidney damage may vary considerably between a small sub-capsular haemorrhage to a rupture involving the whole thickness of the kidney.

Conservative management in the less severe injuries is usually successful and consists of:

Bedrest and Pain relief. The pain may be due to blood clots passing down the ureter.

Blood transfusion may be required for shock and/or if bleeding from the kidney continues.

Intravenous pyelogram is performed as soon as possible to show that the other kidney is functioning normally.

Antibiotic cover is given to prevent any haemotoma from becoming infected.

Regular observation of temperature, pulse and blood pressure.

Examination of all specimens of urine for haematuria.

Regular observation of loin for swelling or bruising which might indicate a perinephric haematoma.

The patient usually remains in bed until haematuria disappears.

In the more severe injuries, surgery may be considered necessary. Pre-operative care obviously depends upon the condition of the patient (who might have multiple injuries) and the time allowed but it usually incorporates the measures mentioned above.

Refer to chapter 1 for General Principles.
The operation would depend upon the extent of damage:
If severely damaged — nephrectomy, partial or complete.

Large single tears may be sutured and a nephrostomy (insertion of a drainage tube) performed.

Smaller tears may be sutured.

It is important that the nursing staff be aware of the details of the operation so that they understand the purpose of the drainage tubes and can prepare the bed area appropriately.

Post-operation — specific nursing care

The patient usually returns to the ward with an intravenous infusion or transfusion in progress which must be maintained according to the prescribed regime.

Serum urea/electrolyte levels will be estimated daily so that adjustments can be made to the i.v. regime.

There may be naso-gastric drainage, this is because the patient who has undergone renal surgery may develop loss of peristalsis with all its consequent problems. Criteria for commencing oral fluids and removing the naso-gastric tube is as for post-gastrointestinal surgery. (See relevant section.)

As soon as his condition allows, he can be supported with pillows in the semi-recumbent position leaning towards his affected side. There may be a wound drainage tube, any drainage fluid must be carefully measured, described and recorded on a fluid balance chart. Any evidence of urine draining via the tube or suture line should be reported at once. The skin may need special attention if this is so. The wound must be carefully observed for bleeding and for swelling or bruising around the loin area. All urine must be accurately measured and the degree of haematuria noted. The patient **may** have an in-dwelling urethral catheter *in situ* and the nurse **may** be asked to record the urinary drainage hourly.

Regular analgesia is given to promote the fullest possible participation of the patient in breathing and limb exercises and regular change of position.

The nursing and post-operative recovery depends very much on whether any other organs were damaged and the general condition of the patient. In uncomplicated cases, one would expect the patient to start mobilizing after 24–48 hours; to resume a normal oral intake within 24–72 hours; to have his wound drainage tube removed when drainage has ceased, usually 48–72 hours; and to have sutures removed from the wound within 7–10 days. Observation of the urine output continues, the amount of urine passed, the presence of any discomfort associated with voiding and the presence of abnormal constituents, particularly blood are all carefully noted.

The importance of an adequate fluid intake is discussed with the patient so that he will continue to drink plenty of fluids after discharge home (usually 10–14 days).

The basic principles of nursing care and management as mentioned above would apply to most operations on the kidney and ureter.

The urinary bladder

The urinary bladder acts as a reservoir for urine, its capacity is considerable, the size of the bladder at any time depends upon the amount of urine it contains.

It lies mostly in the pelvic cavity, but when distended can rise into the abdominal cavity, it lies behind the symphysis pubis and below the small intestine. In the female, it lies in front of the uterus and above the urethra and muscles of the pelvic floor. In the male, it lies in front of the rectum and above the urethra and prostate gland.

The ureters pass obliquely through the bladder wall on either side so that urine is prevented from passing back up the ureters when the bladder contracts.

The walls of the bladder consist of an outer peritoneal layer, a middle muscular, a sub-mucous layer and an inner-mucous membrane of transitional epithelium. The transitional epithelium also lines the ureters. The urethra leaves the bladder inferiorly, its orifice is guarded by a sphincter muscle.

Fig 12 Diagram showing oblique entry of ureter into bladder wall

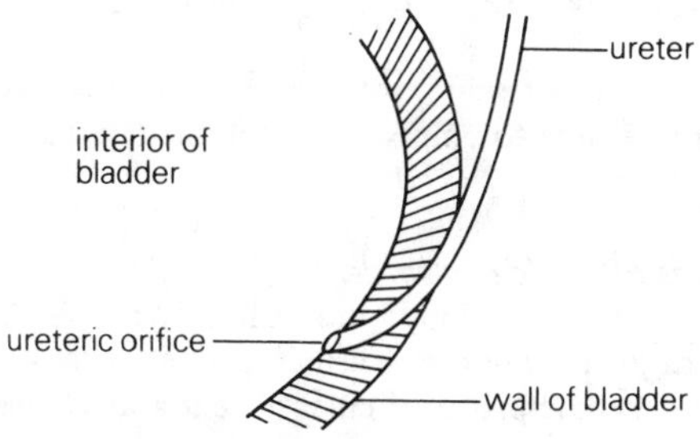

interior of bladder

ureter

ureteric orifice

wall of bladder

Micturition

The voiding of urine is partly a reflex and partly a voluntary act, and disturbances of normal micturition may be indicative of bladder disorder.

The most common disturbances are as follows.

Retention of urine

This may be **acute** or **chronic** and the causes may be many, e.g. after major surgery, due to obstruction to the outflow of urine by stone, prostatic enlargement or urethral stricture. or as a result of injury or disease of the spinal cord.

Alterations in the urinary stream

The patient may have difficulty in starting to micturate, may experience interruptions to the flow or may continue to dribble urine.

Frequency and urgency

The patient may pass small amounts of urine many times during the day and night and this may be accompanied by urgency when the desire to void is sudden and immediate.

Painful micturition

This is termed **dysuria**, the patient complains of pain or burning when voiding, the time and type of pain or discomfort in relation to voiding should be carefully noted.

Incontinence of urine

The patient is unaware or cannot control the passage of urine.

Abnormal constituents

There may be blood, pus or other debris in the urine.

Residual urine

The bladder may not be able to empty itself completely, residual urine will pre-dispose to infection.

Specific investigations of bladder disorder

These would include, history-taking and full physical examination, including palpation of lower abdomen to elicit bladder distension, digital rectal examination to exclude prostatic enlargement and examination of external genitalia to exclude abnormality.

Blood would be taken for full routine tests, particularly urea and electrolyte estimation.

Radiological — Plain abdominal X-rays, intravenous pyelogram, micturating cystogram.

Endoscopic — Cystoscopy and biopsy

Urine testing — ward and laboratory examination

Strict fluid balance recording.

The following are the more common bladder conditions that the nurse might encounter.

Bladder calculi

a Stones may migrate from the kidney and ureter into the bladder where they may obstruct the urethral orifice.

b Stones may form in the bladder itself. These usually result from:
   i conditions which cause stasis of urine and infection
   ii calculi will deposit on any foreign body which might have inadvertently entered the bladder.

The patient may complain of the following:

Pain

In the bladder region, sometimes in the perineum and at the tip of the penis and particularly at the end of micturition. If the stone or particles of stone pass into the urethra, the patient complains of severe pain and possible complete urinary obstruction.

Disturbances of urinary flow — frequency of micturition

Worse during the day probably because in the upright position the stone irritates the sensitive bladder trigone. **Ability to void, only in certain positions,** which are those which keep the stone away from the urethral outlet. **Sudden cessation of flow** before the bladder is emptied which is due to the stone blocking the bladder urethral orifice.

Haematuria

This is caused by irritation of the bladder mucosa by the stone and sometimes this occurs in the last few drops of urine passed. There is frequently accompanying urinary infection.

Types of operation performed

Litholapaxy

The stone(s) is crushed and removed by a special instrument passed through a cystoscope. Pre-operatively, bladder irrigation with an acid solution may have been performed in an attempt to soften the stones.

Suprapubic cystotomy

The bladder is opened through a suprapubic incision and the stone removed. General principles of care and care of drainage will be discussed later but specifically:

The post-operative care involves careful observation of the patient and comparison of symptoms to the pre-operative period. Strict fluid balance recording.

Inspection of all specimens of urine for particles of stone. It may be necessary to irrigate the bladder under the strictest aseptic precautions and to strain the returned fluid for stone debris. An increased fluid intake is needed to wash out the bladder. It is vitally important that the patient is made aware of this and is constantly encouraged to drink plenty.

Bladder trauma

The bladder may be ruptured, as a result of a direct blow to the lower abdomen or as a result of crush injury when it accompanies one or more fractures of the pelvis and possibly injury to other pelvic organs. If the bladder ruptures when it is distended and therefore more vulnerable, it may do so into the peritoneum (intraperitoneal). **Urine leaks into the peritoneal cavity and peritonitis occurs.**

The rupture can also occur extraperitoneally, here the **urine leaks into the surrounding tissues in the pelvis leading to cellulitis and infection**. Leakage of urine from the bladder is termed **extravasation**. Occasionally the bladder may be inadvertently damaged during pelvic operations. If a bladder rupture is suspected, measures would be taken to correct shock and haemorrhage. Whilst caring for the patient during this crucial time the nurse should observe the patient carefully for signs of peritonitis or generalized lower abdominal cellulitis.

A urine specimen should be obtained urgently. If the patient cannot pass urine, the doctor will catheterize the patient. If any difficulty is encountered in passing the catheter, a ruptured urethra may be suspected. The presence of blood is suggestive of injury and a cystogram would be urgently performed to confirm the diagnosis.

The patient would be urgently prepared for surgical repair of the bladder, the bladder would then be drained via a suprapubic catheter and/or urethral catheter until healing of the bladder suture line has occurred. (See care later).

Bladder tumours

These may be **benign** — papilloma or **malignant**

Those tumours which are benign and tend to recur may eventually become malignant.

The patient usually complains of haematuria which is painless and may be intermittent, and sometimes complains of cystitis. However the symptoms will very much depend on whether the tumour is benign or malignant, and if malignant, how advanced the disease is. Investigations would include testing and laboratory examination of urine for analysis, particularly presence of malignant cells. Intravenous pyelogram and cystogram would be done and cystoscopy and biopsy. The treatment would then depend on the diagnosis and extent of the disease process.

Benign papillomatous growths are destroyed by diathermy applied via cystoscopy, subsequently the urine is inspected for the presence of blood for the following 24 hours in hospital after which the patient is discharged home. Fluids must be encouraged after the effects of anaesthesia have worn off.

Many of these patients have a check cystoscopy every 6 months because of the risk of recurrence of growths.

Advice is given to the patient that they should report to their G.P. if they notice any change in their symptoms.

Malignant tumours require more extensive surgery or sometimes radiation and/or chemotherapy or a combination of these treatments. Part or all of the bladder may need to be resected. Partial cystectomy might involve transplantation of one of the ureters while total cystectomy would involve transplantation of both ureters (urinary diversion). A urinary diversion is most commonly achieved by; **formation of ileal conduit** or **ureteroenterostomy**.

Formation of an ileal conduit

This is the transplantation of the ureters into an isolated segment of ileum which is brought out onto the abdominal wall to form an ileostomy spout. Intestinal continuity is maintained.

Pre-operatively, the patient and his family are helped to accept the necessity for the procedure in a similar way to the pre-ileostomy patient. (Refer to relevant section.) His general condition is improved as far as is possible with particular attention to correction of anaemia, fluid and electrolyte imbalance.

The bowel needs to be prepared as for bowel surgery. Urinary antiseptics will be given.

Post-operatively, the patient usually requires a 'special' nurse since the operative procedure will have taken a long time and the patient is likely to be in shock.

General care will be as for post-abdominal surgery. **Only the specific care of the ileal conduit will be discussed here.**

Initially, a catheter may be inserted into the stoma and attached to a closed drainage system. Strict fluid balance is essential and usually the urine output is measured and recorded hourly. **Any cessation of urinary drainage is reported immediately.** Irrigations of the catheter with sterile normal saline may be ordered because of possible obstruction with mucus from the ileal segment.

When the urinary catheter is eventually removed (usually 4–7 days), an ileostomy bag can be fitted over the stoma.

Once his general condition allows, the management of the patient follows that which is necessary to achieve acceptance of the stoma and the fullest degree of self-care which it is possible for the patient to achieve.

Ureteroenterostomy

This involves transplantation of the ureters into the colon thus forming a completely internal diversion. This means that the urine and faeces are eliminated via the same route. The patient learns to control the urine output the same way as he controls defaecation. Urine drains via the ureters into the lower bowel and can be retained until enough accumulates, approx. 200–300 mls, to stimulate the patient as would the defaecation impulse.

The specific problems arising from this procedure post-operatively result from the direct communication of the urinary tract to the bowel (ascending infection to the kidney) and from reabsorption of substances from the accumulating urine via the colon (disturbances of blood chemistry). The patient is advised to void urine every 3–4 hours so that absorption of urinary waste products is minimized.

Strict fluid balance would be necessary initially and correction of any fluid and electrolyte disturbances.

Particular attention would be paid to the skin around the anus and re-assurance and encouragement given to the patient until he can fully control the elimination of urine via his rectum.

General care of the patient would be as for post-abdominal surgery.

Principles of care of patients following bladder surgery

The patient will invariably return to the ward with an intravenous infusion or transfusion in progress. Ensuring an adequate fluid intake is essential to encourage urinary flow. The patient may or may not be allowed to commence oral fluids as soon as the effects of anaesthesia have worn off (this depends on the extent of surgery) so intravenous fluids will need to be continued until such time as the patient can tolerate adequate amounts orally. Encouragement of an adequate oral intake of fluids is one of the nurse's most important functions following specific procedures on the bladder and prostate. If the operative procedure has involved the gastro-intestinal tract, naso-gastric drainage will be *in situ*. (For care see relevant section.) If the bladder has been sutured, there is likely to be a suprapubic drainage tube, this may be as well as an urethral catheter drainage. It is essential that the bladder is not allowed to distend since this would cause tension on the bladder suture line with subsequent leakage of urine and the risk of peritonitis and cellulitis. Drainage is continued until the bladder suture line is healed, for this reason it is important that careful observation is made of all drainage and any sudden cessation reported immediately. It is sometimes necessary to apply suction to the suprapubic tube (because of its position it cannot drain by gravity). Usually this is achieved by means of an electric suction pump the pressure of which can be controlled. It is vitally important that excessive suction is not used as damage to the bladder mucosa can occur. If there is urethral catheter drainage, the catheter may become blocked with blood clot, the tube is then 'milked' to try to dislodge the clot, failing this, bladder irrigation using the strictest aseptic technique is necessary. As mentioned above, adequate fluid intake is most important to flush out the bladder and minimise blockage in all drainages.

As with all other drainage tubes, the security of bladder drainage tubes is important, movement of the patient and attachment of drainage apparatus must be such that there is no 'pull' on any tubing.

Closed drainage systems should not be interrupted unnecessarily, when they need to be, e.g. when changing the collection bag, care must be taken not to introduce infection through to the bladder. In some units it is routine to use collecting bags with taps on the bottom which facilitate emptying and measurement of contents without 'breaking' the closed system.

Special attention is given to the skin around the suprapubic drainage tube as invariably there will be some leakage of urine around the tube with subsequent soreness and possible excoriation of the skin. The skin is cleansed and dried frequently and if an adhesive drainage bag is used over the tube, a good 'seal' should be ensured.

The suprapubic drainage tube is usually removed after 4–7 days, the urethral catheter is left *in situ* for a few days longer in order that the suprapubic opening can heal.

The degree of haematuria is noted daily, catheter specimens of urine may be sent for laboratory examination at any time post-operatively, but one is usually sent routinely prior to removal of catheter.

Removal is best done in early morning so that the patient has all day in which to try to pass urine. If after 8–12 hours no urine has been passed, or if the patient becomes distressed, re-catheterization is necessary. If this happens it is more convenient for all concerned and certainly less distressing for the patient if the procedure is carried out at a reasonable hour and not in the middle of the night. Bladder control is often difficult following removal of the urethral catheter, the patient finds this most distressing, it is wise for one nurse to be responsible in the first few hours at least for reassuring, supporting and supervising his efforts to regain full bladder control. Throughout the period of urinary drainage **strict fluid balance recording is essential**.

General care post-operatively would depend upon the condition of the patient but follows the principles of care following any other major abdominal surgery.

The prostate gland

The prostate gland surrounds the first part of the male urethra as it leaves the bladder. It is described as normally being the size of a chestnut and is encapsulated in fibrous tissue. The substance of the gland is made up of involuntary muscle and glandular epithelium arranged into follicles. Minute ducts open directly into the urethra through which is secreted a fluid which is thought to contribute to the volume of the seminal fluid and increase the mobility of the spermatazoa. The gland is lobulated and is prone to enlargement in the latter part of life. The enlargement may be benign or malignant and the prime feature is that it encroaches on the urinary outlet thus causing disturbance of urinary flow and even complete retention of urine. Stagnant residual urine left in the bladder predisposes to infection.

Management of the patient with retention of urine

The patient is usually admitted in considerable distress. Depending on the length of time since voiding and amount of oral fluid intake, the patient's bladder may range from moderate to gross distension.

Following medical examination, and if his condition allows, the patient is encouraged to void naturally, he may be assisted into the standing position and stimulants such as the noise of running water tried for effect.

If this fails, the patient is catheterized and a closed drainage system established. The bladder is allowed to drain slowly, if the bladder is drained too quickly the sudden drop in intra-abdominal pressure may cause shock and collapse.

Once the patient is made comfortable, investigations into the cause of the retention can begin.

Investigations

Full physical examination including digital rectal examination which will elicit the enlarged prostate gland.

Blood tests would include urea and electrolyte estimation and acid phosphatase estimation (the latter is usually raised in carcinoma of the prostate with metastasis; but blood would either be taken before digital rectal examination or at least 48 hours after, since digital palpation of the prostate causes a transient rise in serum levels).

If abnormal, blood chemistry would be corrected.

Radiological — Intravenous pyelography

Endoscopy — Cystoscopy

Every effort is made to improve the general condition of the patient prior to surgery. Correction of abnormal blood chemistry often improves the 'confused' patient.

Infection is often present and urinary antiseptics are given to remedy this. Oral fluids are encouraged particularly whilst the patient has urethral catheter drainage.

Operations for prostatectomy

Suprapubic prostatectomy

This involves opening the bladder and extracting the gland. Suprapubic drainage or transurethral drainage or both would follow.

Retro-pubic prostatectomy

The bladder is not opened, but the gland approached directly and removed via its capsule which is then repaired. Transurethral drainage would follow and in addition a retro pubic precautionary drain is left *in situ*.

Transurethral prostatectomy

The gland is removed piecemeal via a special cystoscope which carries a diathermy cutting loop which takes pieces out of the prostate. Transurethral drainage follows.

Whilst the patient is in theatre, the bed area is prepared to receive him, the nurse must be aware of the operation performed and wishes of the surgeon in order to have the appropriate urinary drainage apparatus on hand. In addition to the types of drainages already mentioned, the surgeon may request that tidal drainage of the bladder be initiated as soon as the patient returns to the ward. This involves rhythmic filling and draining of the bladder by sterile fluid and if necessary warrants one nurse's attention so that it can be carried out according to the prescribed regime.

The specific care follows the principles discussed in the care of patients following bladder surgery.

Surgery is not always the treatment of choice in carcinoma of the prostate, particularly when the growth is widespread. The patient may need to be treated by radiotherapy and/or chemotherapy (hormone administration).

The urethra

The male urethra is longer than the female's and forms a common pathway for the flow of urine and semen.

It extends from the urinary bladder to the tip of the penis and is described as having three parts, the prostatic urethra, the membranous urethra and the penile portion.

The male urethra sometimes fails to develop completely. Abnormalities include:

meatal stenosis — (narrowing of the external urinary meatus, may be sufficient to cause back-pressure affecting the whole urinary system). Urethral dilatation or surgical repair may be necessary.

hypospadias — the urethra does not extend along the length of the penis so that the external meatus is situated somewhere on the under-surface of the penis or in extreme cases in the perineum. Surgical intervention would depend upon the severity of the condition and may range from simple meatotomy to reconstruction of urethra with temporary urinary diversion. The nursing care would also vary considerably but the main principles of care, as discussed previously, would apply.

Urethral trauma

The membranous portion of the urethra is susceptible to rupture during crush injury to the pelvis with subsequent fractures, and any part of the urethra may be inadvertently damaged by instrumentation.

Surgical repair varies with the degree of trauma, but post-operatively, specifically, would involve care of suprapubic bladder drainage and care of urethral catheter which is perhaps applied to traction until the ruptured urethra heals.

Urethral stricture

This is most often a complication of previous trauma or inflammatory disease. Usually the patient attends hospital at regular intervals for dilatation. It is a relatively simple procedure and because of its regularity, the procedure is known to the patient. Post-operatively, he is encouraged to drink plenty of fluids and the first specimens of urine passed are inspected for blood. Usually the patient is discharged home after 24 hours and a date arranged for follow-up appointment or re-admission.

Practice Questions

Test 6

1. Answer the following questions:
a Which kidney is situated lower than the other and why?
b Name the constituent parts of the nephron.
c What are the three phases of urine formation?
d What is the normal glomerular filtration rate?
e What are the anatomical relations of the male bladder? How do they differ from the female bladder?
f Where is the trigone?
g What are the three functions of urine formation?
h How is urine normally prevented from flowing back up the ureters during micturition?
i What are considered to be the three most common important symptoms of urinary disease?
j What or where is the renal pelvis?
k Where is the prostate gland situated?
l What are considered to be the two specific problems that arise as a result of ureteroenterostomy?
m What is considered to be the normal daily adult urine output?
n Where is the external urethral sphincter?
o What is overflow incontinence?

2. What do you understand by the following terms?
a Hydronephrosis
b Strangury
c Nephrostomy
d Urinary diversion
e Retrograde pyelography
f Dysuria
g Litholopaxy
h Extravasation
i Extraperitoneal bladder rupture
j Ileal conduit
k Retro-pubic prostatectomy
l Hypospadias
m Suprapubic cystostomy
n Transitional epithelium
o Creatinine Clearance Test

3. Mark the following statements true or false:

a Tidal urinary drainage is the total volume of urine passed in 24 hours.

b Swelling in the loin following abdominal injury may be indicative of peri-nephric haematoma.

c Whilst the patient is confined to bed, the urethral drainage collecting bag should not be elevated higher than bed level.

d In acute retention of urine, immediate complete decompression of the bladder is advised following catheterization in order to relieve the patient's discomfort.

e Prolonged severe shock can lead to acute renal failure.

f You may be required to strain all specimens of urine passed following litholopaxy.

g You would not expect leakage of urine around a subrapubic cystotomy drainage tube.

h You would not expect leakage of urine around a nephrostomy tube.

i Sudden cessation of urinary flow before the patient feels the bladder is emptied may be indicative of bladder calculus.

j Digital rectal examination may cause a lowering of the serum acid phosphatase levels.

k You would normally expect suprapubic bladder drainage following transurethral prostatectomy.

l Scrotal and penile swelling following a fractured pelvis might be due to superficial extravasation of urine from a ruptured urethra.

Answers to Test 6

1.

a The right kidney is usually situated lower than the left due to the space taken up by the liver.

b Glomerulus — Bowman's capsule — proximal convoluted tubule — Loop of Henle — distal convoluted tubule — collecting tubule.

c Glomerular filtration — selective tubular re-absorption — tubular secretion.

d 120 mls/minute.

e The male bladder lies behind the symphysis pubis, in front of the rectum and seminal vesicles, below the small intestine and above the urethra and prostate gland. The female bladder has the same structures in front and above it, but lies in front of the uterus and above the urethra and muscles of the pelvic floor.

f The triangular area situated between the ureteric and urethral orifices in the bladder.

g Maintenance of water balance, electrolyte balance and pH of blood.

h By compression of the bladder walls on the obliquely inserted ureters.

i Pain, frequency of micturition and haematuria.

j The renal pelvis refers to the upper expanded end of the ureter.

k The prostate surrounds the commencement of the urethra as it leaves the bladder.

l Ascending infection to the kidney and disturbances of blood chemistry.

m About 1,500 mls in 24 hours.

n The external urethral sphincter is situated at the distal end of the prostatic urethra.

o It is the term sometimes given to the frequent voiding or dribbling of small amounts of urine as a result of retention of urine and a distended bladder.

2.

a Dilatation of the pelvis and distension of the kidney due to obstruction in the ureter.

b Extreme pain accompanied by the need to micturate but resulting in the expulsion of only a small amount of blood stained urine.

c Tube or catheter drainage through the body of the kidney.

d Surgically diverting the flow of urine away from its normal channel. It may be a temporary or permanent measure.

e Introduction of a radio-opaque substance into ureteric catheters that have been inserted via a cystoscope.

f Pain or discomfort experienced during micturition.

g Crushing and removal of bladder calculi by means of a lithotrite passed via cystoscopy.

h Leakage of urine from some point in the urinary tract into the surrounding tissues.

i Usually involves rupture of the lower end of the bladder outside the peritoneum.

j Transplantation of ureters into an isolated segment of ileum which is brought out to the abdominal wall (urinary diversion). The intestinal continuity is maintained.

k Direct approach to the prostate which is excised via its capsule. The bladder is therefore not opened.

l Developmental abnormality of the urethra which opens onto the under surface of the penis or into the perineum.

m Opening and tube drainage of the bladder through the lower abdominal wall.

n The special epithelial lining only found in the urinary tract.

o Involves 24 hour collection of urine and venous blood specimens for creatinine concentration estimation. The volume of plasma cleared of creatinine per minute should be equal to the glomerular filtration rate.

3.

a	False	e	True	i	True
b	True	f	True	j	False
c	True	g	False	k	False
d	False	h	True	l	True

8 THE TRACHEA AND THORAX

The objectives of this section are to state:

1 The regional and applied anatomy and physiology of the trachea and respiratory tract.
2 The pre- and post- operative care after tracheostomy and thoracic surgery.

Respiration

The functions of breathing are as follows.

1 To take in oxygen which is needed by all the cells of the body for the oxidation of foodstuffs and the production of heat and energy.
2 To give off carbon dioxide which is the waste product of the above process.
3 By regulating the carbon dioxide levels in the blood, breathing helps maintain the blood pH at 7.4 which is slightly alkaline.

The processes which facilitate the above functions are:

a **ventilation**
b **diffusion**
c **perfusion**

Ventilation

This is the movement of:

i air rich in oxygen from the atmosphere, through the respiratory passages, into the alveoli
ii alveolar air rich in carbon dioxide back through the respiratory passages into the atmosphere

This movement depends upon **the patency of the respiratory passages,** the pharynx, larynx, trachea, bronchi, bronchioles; **an intact chest wall** which provides an airtight box and **the integrity of the nerves and muscles** which bring about an increase and decrease in the size of the thoracic cavity.

Respiration is controlled by the **respiratory centre** in the medulla of the brain. The pH of blood and levels of carbon dioxide in the blood are two important influences on the activity of this centre. Impulses pass via nerves from the respiratory centre to the anterior horn cells of the spinal cord from where the phrenic nerves arise from cervical roots to supply the diaphragm, and intercostal nerves arise from thoracic roots to supply the external intercostal muscles. These are known as the inspiratory muscles, inspiration being an **active process.**

The size of the thoracic cavity is increased when the diaphragm contracts downwards and the rib cage swings upwards and outwards. This increases the negative pleural pressure and the lungs which are covered by the visceral and parietal pleura, expand, thus drawing air from the atmosphere.

Expiration, a **passive process** is brought about by the elastic recoil of the lungs and relaxation of the inspiratory muscles, this increases the pleural pressure and air is forced out into the atmosphere.

Diffusion

The exchange of oxygen from the alveoli into the blood in the pulmonary capillaries and carbon dioxide from the blood into the alveoli. Diffusion depends upon:

a the difference in the 'tension' (partial pressures) of the gases across membranes,

b the area and thickness of the alveolar/capillary membrane,

a Oxygen passes from the alveolar air into the blood in the pulmonary capillaries because the tension in the alveolar air is greater than in the blood. Carbon dioxide moves in the opposite direction. At tissue level oxygen passes from the blood to the tissue fluid, then to the cells because the oxygen tension is higher in the blood than in the tissues. Carbon dioxide tension is higher in the cells than in the blood so moves from the cells and tissues into the blood.

b The alveoli are lined with flattened epithelium and are in close proximity to numerous capillaries through the walls of which diffusion of gases can take place. Normally ventilation of the alveoli and perfusion (flow of blood) are balanced. — **ventilation — perfusion ratio.** A disturbance in this ratio can result in **under-ventilation or under-perfusion.** Diffusion may also be decreased by changes in the alveolar tissue resulting from chronic lung disease.

Perfusion

This is the circulation of blood through the pulmonary capillaries where diffusion takes place — **external or pulmonary respiration** — and the circulation of blood to all the tissues of the body where **internal** or **tissue respiration** takes place.

Relevant anatomy

The upper respiratory passages, — nose, pharynx, — which are lined with highly vascular mucous membrane serve to warm and humidify the air as it is breathed in. Hairs in the nose, sticky with mucus, have a filtering effect, trapping particles in the inspired air.

The larynx is protected by the epiglottis during swallowing, thus preventing food from entering the airway. The larynx is comprised of a number of irregular shaped cartilages and contains the vocal cords. It is one of the organs involved in speech but is not essential since post-laryngectomy patients can be taught oesophageal speech.

The trachea extends from a level of C6 above to T5 below, where it bifurcates to become the left and right bronchi.

The lower part of the trachea is in close proximity to the major blood vessels leaving the heart, the bifurcation of the trachea being pushed to the right by the arch of the aorta.

The patency of the trachea is maintained by the C-shaped rings of hyaline cartilage found in the outer covering of its wall. These cartilages are connected to one another by fibrous and elastic tissue. The blood vessels, nerves and lymphatics are found in the middle connective tissue layer. The inner layer is composed of ciliated epithelium containing goblet cells.

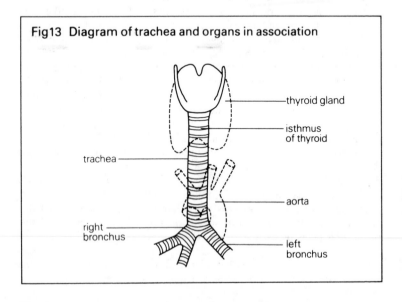

Fig 13   Diagram of trachea and organs in association

thyroid gland

isthmus of thyroid

trachea

aorta

right bronchus

left bronchus

Tracheostomy

The trachea forms part of the respiratory passages, the function of which is to warm, moisten and filter the air that is breathed in. In quiet breathing about 400 ml of air is breathed in and out, known as **tidal volume**. However only the first 250 ml of the air reaches the alveoli, the remaining 150 ml occupies the respiratory passages. This 150 ml is referred to as **dead space air**. This means that the first 150 ml of each expiration is dead space air, it is only the last 250 ml of each expiration which contains alveolar air.

This means that:

a some of the effort in breathing is to take in air that never reaches the lungs,

b if for any reason the tidal volume falls, less air reaches the lungs because 150 ml of air will always be needed to occupy the dead space.

Reasons for tracheostomy (an opening into the trachea).

1 **To relieve obstruction of the upper respiratory passages** — air is breathed directly into the trachea thus bypassing the obstruction.

2 **To alleviate respiratory distress** — a tracheostomy reduces the dead space thus allowing air to reach the lungs with less respiratory effort.

3 **To allow better access to pulmonary secretions** which cannot be effectively expectorated — more effective suction can be performed via the tracheostomy.

4 **To allow mechanically assisted ventilation** in cases of respiratory paralysis or inefficiency when an airtight connection is necessary to prevent loss of ventilatory gas. Although this can be effected by means of an endotracheal tube, a tracheostomy is usually considered after 48 hours.

5 **As a preliminary procedure** to certain operations in the neck region.

Pre-operative

The specific preparation of the patient will depend very much on the reasons why the procedure is considered necessary. In some instances it needs to be carried out as an emergency procedure, in others, there would be more time for preparation.

Where time allows as perhaps when the planned tracheostomy is a preliminary to an extensive throat operation, the aim would be to render the patient as fit as possible for surgery thus preparing him physically and psychologically for the outcome of the operation and/or tracheostomy. Another obvious important consideration would be whether tracheostomy is to be permanent or temporary.

In the 'intensive care' situation the patient might be neither well enough nor alert enough to consider the implications of the procedure.

Operation
The isthmus of the thyroid is free from the trachea and divided. This exposes the upper three or four tracheal rings. A segment of the second and third rings is excised and a tracheostomy tube inserted, the skin is closed around it.

The ward area is specifically prepared for the patient's return.

Post-operative
General considerations: The patient would be received back into a ward area where he could be constantly observed. An experienced nurse should be in attendance. Usually the patient would be nursed in an 'intensive care' situation.

The general care would depend upon a number of factors e.g. the reason why the tracheostomy was necessary, the patient's level of consciousness, the extent and nature of the operative procedure, the site of wounds and drainage tubes and whether the patient is breathing independently or not, to mention but a few.

The position in which the patient would be nursed would also depend upon the above factors, but generally, if the patient is conscious, he is sat up well-supported by pillows as soon as his condition allows.

Specific care of the tracheostomy
As soon as the patient is returned to bed the nurse should check:
a the type of tube *in situ*
b the security of the tube
c the patency of the tube
d the position of the tube
e the wound site
and thereafter at frequent intervals.

a The type of tube *in situ*
Usually, either a metal type which consists of three or four separate parts, an outer tube which is usually not removed, an introducer, an inner tube which can be removed frequently for cleaning and can be used alternately with a speaking tube **or** a portex cuffed tube which is usually not removed.

It is sometimes necessary to change the outer metal tube or portex cuffed tube because of obstruction due to accumulation of secretions. Should this be necessary during the first few days following operation the tube is changed by a doctor or trained nurse, tracheal dilators being used to keep the tracheostomy track open until the new tube is inserted.

After the first few weeks the tracheostomy track becomes well-established and tubes can be changed/removed without fear of the wound edges being sucked in on inspiration or closing up.

b The security of the tube

To prevent the tube being coughed out or accidently removed it is secured in position by means of paired tapes tied around the neck. The ties should be tied at the side of the neck allowing easy access for the nurse, she should check that the tapes are not tied too tightly.

c The patency of the tube

The tube or trachea may become blocked with mucus. In the first few days **frequent suction** is needed to remove this, this can be distressing for the patient and the nurse should familiarize herself with the special technique to be used. She must take every precaution in order to:

   i not introduce infection into the bronchi

   ii prevent trauma (bronchial ulceration) to the bronchial lining by over zealous technique.

When a metal tube is *in situ,* the inner tube can be removed when necessary, cleaned and put back (see above for change of tube). As soon as the patient can co-operate, deep breathing exercises and expectoration are encouraged, the physiotherapist visits the patient frequently. This intensive physiotherapy, together with antibiotic cover is to reduce the risk of pulmonary infection and collapse. The patient is reluctant to cough initially, often being frightened that he will cough out the tube. Patience, supervision, encouragement and reassurance are essential to allay the patients fears.

Humidification

The normal function of the upper air passages is to warm, filter and moisten the air. This function is lost when a tracheostomy is performed, there is thus a danger of drying and crusting of secretions which may lead to obstruction.

Various attachments are available to help overcome this problem. The nurse should be aware of the wishes of the doctor in charge. If the patient needs assisted ventilation, the machines usually have 'built in' humidifiers. If the patient is breathing naturally, measures may range between the following.

a Simply covering the tracheostomy tube with a large single layer square of moistened gauze, this also lessens the risk of inhalation of foreign particles. The gauze piece should be changed frequently, it should not be allowed to become saturated with mucus.

b Attachment of tracheostomy tube to a humidifier with or without oxygen.

c Use of various preparations e.g. Alevaire.

The position of the tube

The neck wound is usually protected by a light keyhole gauze dressing which is placed under the diaphragm of the tracheostomy tube. The nurse should check that the diaphragm is positioned flat against the dressing. If it is not lying flat there is the possibility of tracheal pressure necrosis.

Possible causes of a badly placed tube:

i short tube — it is possible for the tube to come out of the trachea but still appear to be in position, the nurse should observe the neck for swelling and surgical emphysema;

ii tapes tied too tightly — thus pulling the tube against the wall of the trachea, this will eventually lead to ulceration and necrosis;

iii dragging on the tube — by attachment tubing from ventilator or humidification apparatus.

Tracheal ulceration can also be produced by over-inflation of the cuff of the portex tube. Great care is taken to avoid this, the nurse may be asked to deflate the cuff for 2 minutes every hour following pharyngeal suction. Tracheal stenosis may occur as a late complication of tracheal ulceration/necrosis.

Other specific nursing points

Wound care

The wound will require frequent toilet and change of keyhole dressing because of contamination by mucus.

Sutures are removed 5–8 days.

Loss of voice

This can be distressing for the patient and reassurance will be according to whether the tracheostomy is permanent or temporary. Whilst the patient is unable to speak, the nurse call system should be at hand together with a pen, writing pad, and communication cards. If the tracheostomy is permanent, speech therapy is commenced as soon as the patient's condition warrants.

Dysphagia
If the patient is conscious, he may complain of difficulty in swallowing. Encouragement of oral fluids and a soft diet is necessary until this improves.

Practice Questions

Test 7

1. Answer the following questions:

a What is/are the function(s) of breathing?

b Describe the processes which facilitate breathing.

c Where is the respiratory centre situated?

d What are the main inspiratory muscles called?

e Give the reasons why a tracheostomy may be performed.

f Which part of the respiratory cycle is a passive process? Explain.

g Which organ lies immediately posteriorly to the trachea?

h How is the patency of the trachea normally maintained?

i Briefly describe how the wall of the trachea is structured.

j List the most common causes of tracheal obstruction.

k What are the functions of the upper respiratory passages?

l What is the anatomical relationship of the trachea to the thyroid gland?

m List the specific observations that should be made of the tracheostomy in the post-operative period.

n Why is it important to observe whether the diaphragm of the tube lies flat to the patient's neck?

2. What do you understand by the following terms?

a Perfusion

b Tidal volume

c Dead space air

d Diffusion

e Ventilation

f External respiration

g Blood pH

h Surgical emphysema

i Pressure necrosis (tracheal)

j Vital capacity

k Tissue (internal) respiration

l Tracheal suction

m Tracheal dilator

n Asphyxia

3. Mark the following statements true or false:

a The tracheal cartilages keep the trachea patent in all positions of the neck.

b One of the advantages of a tracheostomy is to increase the dead space.

c   Tracheal suction is best performed during the inspiratory phase.

d   Pharyngeal suction is advised immediately prior to tracheostomy tube cuff deflation.

e   During the first 48 hours post-operatively the portex type (one-piece) tracheostomy tube should be removed frequently by the nurse for cleaning.

f   Continuous tracheal suction may be necessary for very tenacious secretions.

g   Over-inflation of the tracheostomy tube cuff causes pressure necrosis of the tracheal mucosa.

h   Dragging of the tracheostomy tube downwards (e.g. by ventilator attachment tubes) may lead to posterior tracheal wall damage.

i   Marked respiratory effort not relieved by suctioning should be reported immediately.

j   Swelling of the neck and face may be caused by leakage of air into the subcutaneous tissues around the tracheostomy.

Answers to Test 7

1. **a**   i   to take in oxygen
         ii   to give out carbon dioxide
        iii   the regulation of blood pH.

   b   i   Ventilation — movement of air in and out of the chest.
         ii   Diffusion — the passage and interchange of oxygen and carbon dioxide through the alveolar/capillary membranes.
        iii   Perfusion — the circulation of blood through capillaries where exchange of gases can take place.

   c   In the medulla of the brain.

   d   External intercostal muscles, diaphragm.

   e   i   to relieve upper respiratory obstruction
         ii   to reduce anatomical dead space
        iii   to facilitate easier suctioning
         iv   to allow mechanically assisted ventilation
          v   as a preliminary to neck operations.

   f   Expiration — due to the elastic recoil of living tissue and relaxation of intercostal muscles and diaphragm.

   g   Oesophagus.

   h   By the C-shaped rings of hyaline cartilage.

   i   Outer fibrous, middle connective, inner mucous membrane with goblet cells.

   j   i   Impaction of foreign body
         ii   Acute infections and oedema

    iii Tumours

    iv Stenosis following scalding

     v Paralysis of vocal cords

    vi Cut throat

k To warm, filter and moisten the inspired air.

l The isthmus which connects the two lobes of the thyroid gland lies over the front of the upper part of the trachea.

m The type, security, patency and position of the tube and the wound site.

n A badly positioned tube may cause pressure necrosis of the tracheal mucosa.

2.

a Circulation of blood through to the capillaries where exchange of gases can take place.

b Volume of air breathed in and out in quiet respiration.

c Volume of air which occupies the airways in breathing.

d The passage and exchange of gases $CO_2 + CO_2$ from a high pressure to a low pressure through the semi-permeable membranes.

e Movement of air in and out of the chest.

f Exchange of $O_2 + CO_2$ through the alveolar and pulmonary capillary membranes.

g The reaction of blood is slightly alkaline 7.4 pH.

h Collection of air in the subcutaneous tissues.

i Unrelieved pressure on the tracheal mocosal lining interferes with the blood supply to that area resulting in death of tissue.

j The amount of air breathed. The largest possible inspiration is followed by the largest possible expiration.

k The exchange of $O_2 + CO_2$ between blood and the cells.

l A method of removal of secretions from the trachea and bronchis, can be performed via endoscopy, endotracheal tube or tracheostomy.

m An instrument used to keep the tracheostomy track open, if the tracheostomy tube is accidently pulled or coughed out. It is a life-saving measure in the early post-operative period.

n A state where there is insufficient oxygen in the blood **accompanied** by an accumulation of carbon dioxide (as would occur in obstruction or drowning for example) and where the person would fight for breath.

3.

a	True	**e**	False	**h**	True
b	False	**f**	False	**i**	True
c	False	**g**	True	**j**	True
d	True				

The thorax — relevant A/P

Pulmonary ventilation depends upon the patency of the respiratory airways, an intact chest wall and the integrity of the nerves and muscles which bring about an increase and decrease in the size of the thoracic cavity.

The skeletal framework of the thorax is formed by the sternum anteriorly, the thoracic vertebrae posteriorly, and the remainder of the circumference by the ribs. The diaphragm is the dome shaped muscle which separates the thoracic from the abdominal cavity. The thorax **acts as an airtight box** in which are situated the two lungs and **in which pressure can be varied** by altering the size of the thoracic cavity.

The lungs almost fill the thoracic cavity, they are separated from each other by the mediastinum in which are found the heart and major blood vessels.

The rt. and lt. bronchi enter the corresponding lungs and divide and sub-divide into smaller branches, the terminal branches being referred to as bronchioles. Like the trachea, **the patency of these airways must be ensured.** The walls of the larger bronchi are structured similarly to the trachea but the cartilage in the smaller bronchi is found as irregular plates which become smaller and fewer in number with each successive branching. The walls of the bronchioles are composed of smooth muscle lined with mucous membrane. There are no goblet cells and the cartilage is absent. The smooth muscle fibres, which have a vagal and sympathetic nerve supply, are arranged circularly and their construction causes narrowing of the lumen of the bronchioles.

The bronchi and all but the finest bronchioles serve merely as airways. The lung tissue proper consists of **lung units** each composed of a terminal bronchiole supplying a cluster of air spaces called alveoli.

The walls of the alveoli are composed of a single layer of cells and are surrounded by a network of blood capillaries. It is through this alveolar-

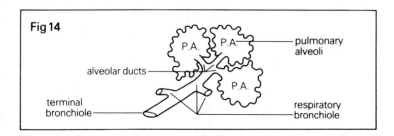

Fig 14

pulmonary alveoli

alveolar ducts

P.A.   P.A.

P.A.

terminal bronchiole

respiratory bronchiole

capillary membrane that the interchange of gases takes place. (See ventilation-perfusion ratio — last chapter).

Branches of each bronchus are accompanied by branches of the pulmonary artery, this 'matching' arrangement supply segments of lung tissue. Knowledge of the segmental arrangement is essential in the understanding of treatment of lung disease e.g. bronchial obstruction, postural drainage etc.

Drainage of the lung segments is via the pulmonary veins. The lung tissue itself is supplied with oxygenated blood via the bronchial arteries.

Each lung is invested in a double serous membrane called the **pleura.** The **parietal pleura** lines the interior of the chest wall and upper surface of the diaphragm. It folds back at the root of the lung (where the bronchi and blood vessels enter and leave the lung) to form the **visceral pleura** which completely enclose the lung except at its root.

These two surfaces are separated by a small amount of serous fluid which acts as a lubricant, allowing the pleural surfaces to glide over each other during lung movements.

There is no gap between the two pleural surfaces normally but there is a **potential space** which is termed the **pleural cavity.**

The pressure between the layers of pleura (and throughout the thorax) is less than in the atmosphere. This is due to **the elasticity** of the lungs. Each time the thorax is expanded, the pressure within the air-sacs is reduced, thus atmospheric air enters through the patent airways to equalize the pressure. Each time the lungs expand, the elastic tissue is stretched, this tissue has a tendency to recoil back to its original size, this pulling effect

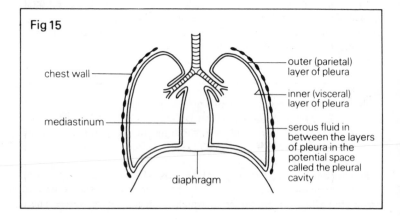

Fig 15

chest wall

mediastinum

diaphragm

outer (parietal) layer of pleura

inner (visceral) layer of pleura

serous fluid in between the layers of pleura in the potential space called the pleural cavity of the lungs away from the walls of the thorax cannot separate the layers of pleura and a 'negative' pressure is created within the pleural cavity.

If sufficient air or fluid collects between the pleural surfaces, as may occur from a ruptured bullae or an open wound in the chest wall or following thoracic surgery, it will prevent the underlying lung from expanding and cause lung collapse. Unrelieved, it may also cause pressure on and displacement of the heart and blood vessels (mediastinal shift) and eventually pressure on the unaffected lung. If this occurred there would be circulatory and respiratory embarrassment.

Patients in need of major thoracic surgery are usually referred to specialized thoracic units, similarly, accident victims whose injuries include thoracic injuries may be nursed on an intensive care unit. Nevertheless, in the general ward, procedures may be carried out in which

a **the pleural space is deliberately entered** e.g. thoracic surgical operations on the chest wall and on structures inside the thorax.

Transthoracic operations where the surgeon opens the chest to gain wider access to organs in the upper abdomen e.g. on the diaphragm, oesophagus or stomach.

b **the pleural space may be inadvertently opened** operations or procedures in lower part of neck e.g. thyroidectomy; in region of diaphragm e.g. nephrectomy; on chest wall e.g. mastectomy.

When the pleural vacuum space is entered (deliberately or inadvertently or as a result of penetrating wound or crush injury), a state of **pneumothorax** or **haemothorax** or both exists. If this happens on one side, the patient is dependent on greater expansion of the opposite lung. Unrelieved, it may produce mediastinal shift and eventual embarrassment of the opposite lung. If pneumothorax occurs on both sides, interference with lung expansion may be such as to produce asphyxia and death.

Under-water seal drainage

One of the special features of nursing patients who have undergone thoracic operations is the need for, and care associated with, the closed chest drainage apparatus or **underwater seal drainage.**

The purpose of the underwater seal drainage is to restore the pleural vacuum or 'negative' pressure by facilitating the escape of air or fluid from the pleural cavity which, if allowed to accumulate would prevent the lung from expanding.

A large tube is inserted through the chest wall. The outer end of the tube is not left open but connected to tubing the other end of which is inserted into a sterile bedside container in which is placed sterile water. There must be sufficient water in the bottle to cover the end of the tube to a 5–8 cm depth, but no more.

As the patient breathes in, the vacuum created pulls water up the tube of the underwater seal, but the weight of the water column prevents it being drawn up the tube more than a few centimetres. This preserves the vacuum in the pleural cavity and allows the lung to expand. At the same time any drainage fluid can escape down the tube into the bedside bottle. **Air escapes from the pleural cavity on expiration but cannot be sucked back through the water seal on inspiration.**

There may be a need for more than one drainage tube when there is both air and fluid in the pleural cavity.

It is occasionally necessary to attach a suction apparatus to the underwater seal bedside apparatus. See chapter 2 Fig. 4.

Pre-operation

As well as the general principles of pre-operative preparation that apply to all patients undergoing surgery, the following are additional important considerations regarding the preparation of patients for thoracic surgery or if a transthoracic approach to the abdominal cavity is anticipated.

The patient may require an extended pre-operative preparation in order to

1   improve his hydration and nutritional status
2   carry out investigative/evaluation procedures
3   correct any conditions which may predispose to post-operative complications.

1 Improve his hydration and nutritional status.

It may be possible to improve the patient's nutritional status by encouraging him to take a high calorie diet with increased proteins and vitamins. However, the patient's appetite may be poor or condition such that he is unable to swallow, or unable to tolerate an increased intake. Depending on the underlying condition for which surgery is indicated:

a   the diet may be liquidized and supplemented with commercial concentrates which can be added to fluids of the patient's choice,
b   the diet may be given via naso-gastric tube,
c   in the more extreme cases, the required calories, electrolytes and fluids may be given via the intravenous route.

Ensuring a satisfactory state of hydration helps in the removal of pulmonary secretions.

2 carry out investigative/evaluation procedures

The initial investigations may have included:

a   radiological studies — e.g. chest X-ray, bronchogram, pulmonary angiography,

b   endoscopic studies — e.g. laryngoscopy, bronchoscopy and biopsy,

c   lung function tests — e.g. measurement of lung volumes.

All previous investigative results should be available.

Nearer to the time for surgery, a chest X-ray is likely to be repeated and ECG would be performed.

Blood tests (routine) plus arterial blood gas levels would be estimated.

Sputum specimens would be sent for analysis, culture and sensitivity test.

3 correct any conditions which may predispose to post-operative complications

This, of course, applies to all patients undergoing all types of surgery. The nurse should use the time to observe her patient carefully and give appropriate advice where necessary, in order that any potential problems can be identified as early as possible.

During this pre-operative period, the nurse should note the following:

a   Temperature

b   Pulse — rate, rhythm and volume

c   Respirations — rate, rhythm, depth, character, a description of chest movements may also be asked for.

d   Blood pressure

e   Exercise tolerance

f   Amount and characteristics of sputum — consistency, colour, whether purulent.

g   Presence and characteristics of cough.

Pre-operative chest physiotherapy is obviously vitally important. Depending on the patient's condition this might range from regular deep breathing exercises and expectoration, through to intensive therapy including chest percussion and vibration techniques and postural drainage. Antibiotic therapy is likely to be prescribed.

The aims of chest physiotherapy — pre-operative

a   To improve the efficiency of ventilation.

b   To clear excessive secretions.

c   To mobilize all the joints involved in breathing and help improve the patient's posture.

d   To explain and teach post-operative exercises and the patient's role in performing them.

The aims of chest physiotherapy — post-operative
a To maintain the above.
b To prevent lung and circulatory complications.
c To maintain the efficiency of unaffected areas of the lung.
d To re-expand affected areas of the lung.
e To increase exercise tolerance.

Whilst the patient is undergoing surgery, the area in the ward to which he will return is prepared.

Particular attention should be paid to the provision of appropriate suction and oxygen equipment. In addition:

Equipment to facilitate underwater seal (closed) drainage.

Two large clamp forceps.

Central venous pressure measurement might be required.

The nursing staff should be able to obtain equipment for emergency re-insertion of chest drain and chest aspiration should it be required.

Post-operation
Positioning
The usual criteria for positioning the patient applies (see chapter 1) but there are additional measures to be taken.

The head end of the bed **may be elevated slightly,** this helps the patient's breathing by lowering the diaphragm. The patient should be turned every 1–2 hours, instructions will be received from the surgeon as to the specific position(s) he wishes for the patient, each position should be such that full expansion of the unaffected lung is allowed. This means that generally, the patient can be nursed on his back, inclined towards and on his affected side.

Any movement of the patient should be preceded by clamping of the drainage tubes above the connection and lifting of the tubes during the move to prevent them dragging. When the patient is comfortably positioned, the clamps are removed and the drainage apparatus checked for patency. **All moves and lifts should be carefully thought through before they begin, to ensure the comfort and safety of the patient and maintenance of patency of all drainage apparatus.**

Continuous oxygen therapy may be prescribed for the first 12–24 hours, the patient's need for O_2 will be assessed in relation to level and stability of vital signs and arterial blood gas levels and pH.

Nursing observations and care

1 Maintenance of prescribed intravenous regime.
2 Central venous pressure recordings $\frac{1}{2}$–1 hourly initially, this might be necessary to show:
a the extent to which the rt. side of the heart is coping with a reduction in the pulmonary circulation when a lung or part of a lung has been resected
b how the respiratory movements and changes in intrathoracic pressure is affecting the venous return to the heart.
3 Colour and texture of skin and comparison of trunk with extremities.
4 Initially, $\frac{1}{4}$–1 hourly recordings of
a Pulse — rate, rhythm and volume.
b Respirations — rate, rhythm, depth and sounds, observe for equal movements both sides of chest, abnormal movements of intercostal spaces and involvement of the accessory muscles of respiration (muscles of shoulder girdle and abdomen).
c Pulmonary Function Tests — tidal volume, minute volume and forced expiratory volume being the most usual.
d Blood Pressure — $\frac{1}{2}$–1 hourly initially
e Temperature — 1–2 hourly
5 Wound area — check for bleeding
   Chest drainage apparatus — check for security and patency
6 If the operative procedure has involved the gastro-intestinal tract: observation and care of naso-gastric drainage, abdominal wound and perhaps abdominal tube.

The frequency of recording of observations would be adjusted in response to changes in the patient's condition.

Pain relief

It is essential for the comfort of the patient and to ensure his fullest co-operation in moving and regular change of position and his participation in the intensive post-operative chest physiotherapy, that the patient's pain should be kept to a minimum.

Regular analgesia is prescribed and given. The narcotic group of drugs tend not to be used because of their respiratory depressive action. It is essential that the patient **coughs to remove secretions** and **breathes deeply** to ventilate all parts of the lungs.

Fluids/nutrition

If the operation has not involved the gastro-intestinal tract, the patient **may** be allowed small amounts of clear oral fluids as soon as the effects of the anaesthetic have worn off. These can be increased gradually as tolerated and a light diet may be commenced in the first 1-2 days. Intravenous fluids are usually continued at least for the first 48 hours.

Wound care

The wound would normally not require any special attention other than the specific care associated with the drainage tube.

Sutures would be removed in 10-14 days.

Chest X-rays would be performed daily before and following removal of the drainage tubes to check lung expansion.

Exercise/mobilization/rehabilitation programme

In the immediate post-operative period, the patient's position is changed frequently. Intensive chest physiotherapy is initiated and continued until the patient is fully ambulant.

Initially passive limb exercises may be carried out but as soon as the patient's condition improves, he is encouraged to perform active exercise. He may be assisted out of bed as early as the 2nd or 3rd day, this depends on the surgeon and the condition of the patient. Early ambulation lessens the risk of circulatory complications, improves respiratory function, is a welcome postural change from bedrest and serves to boost the patient psychologically. Great care needs to be taken if the chest drainage tubes are still *in situ*.

As the patient's condition improves and particularly after removal of the drainage tubes, activity is increased. It is important to note the patient's response to this, so that his rehabilitative programme can be adjusted in accordance with his exercise tolerance. The convalescent period is usually a lengthy one and consideration has to be given as to whether the patient can return to his normal life pattern, or whether some adaptations need to be made.

Support and advice from the medical, nursing and support services is essential if the patient is to return to the highest possible level of independence.

Practice questions

Test 8

Answer the following questions:

1. **a** List the boundaries of the thoracic cavity.
   b What structures separate the two lungs?
   c i In what ways do the structure of the walls of the bronchioles differ from the bronchi?
       ii the trachea?
   d How many lobes has each lung?
   e Briefly outline the circulation of blood between the right atrium and the left ventricle.
   f Which vessels supply the lung tissue itself with oxygenated blood?
   g Differentiate between the covering of the lungs.
   h Briefly describe the oxygen and carbon dioxide exchange through the alveolar capillary membrane.
   i What are the air sacs?
   j What is the purpose of clamping the chest drainage tube near to the chest when moving the patient?
   k What are the two most important rules regarding the positioning of the bedside drainage bottle (underwater seal)?
   l What is the purpose of the underwater seal drainage?

What do you understand by the following terms?

2. **a** Pleural cavity
   b Double serous membrane
   c Potential space
   d Pneumothorax
   e Mediastinal shift
   f Lung unit
   g Exercise tolerance
   h Accessary muscles of respiration
   i Ventilation/perfusion ratio
   j Postural drainage
   k Paradoxical breathing
   l Minute volume
   m Water seal chest drainage
   n Dyspnoea
   o Pleural effusion

Mark the following statements true or false

3. a Following thoracic surgery, the patient should be positioned leaning towards his unaffected lung, thus leaving the affected lung uppermost to encourage expansion.

   b Blockage of the chest drainage tube would be indicated by an oscillating fluid level in the underwater drainage system.

   c The bedside drainage bottle of the underwater seal system should be changed each time the total fluid level exceeds 8–10 cm above the end of the insertion drainage tube.

   d When changing the underwater seal drainage bottle, the total volume of fluid in the bedside bottle constitutes the patient's fluid loss and is entered on the fluid balance chart.

   e Coughing is discouraged until the chest drainage tubes are removed, when intensive chest physiotherapy can begin.

   f The first thing the nurse should do if the chest drainage becomes disconnected is to position the patient comfortably, reassure him, move the bedside drainage bottle where it cannot be knocked over and inform Sister at once.

   g If the drainage tube is accidently pulled out of the chest, the nurse should seal the wound immediately.

   h A combination of air, sputum and blood are likely to drain via the underwater seal drainage system.

   i Observations during the early post-operative period include the frequency, rhythm and depth of respirations. Use of the accessary respiratory muscles would be normal in a patient with a closed chest drainage.

   j Venous blood samples would be taken daily in order to estimate blood gas levels.

Answers to test 8

1.

a Sternum anteriorly, vertebral column posteriorly, the rest of circumference by the ribs and intercostal muscles, the diaphragm below and the organs forming the root of the neck above.

b The structures in the mediastinum, heart and major vessels, trachea and bronchi, other nerves, blood vessels and glands.

c The trachea has C-shaped rings of cartilage and mucosal goblet cells, the bronchi have irregular plates of cartilage which get fewer and smaller with successive branching. The bronchioles are composed of smooth muscle lined with mucous membranes.

No goblet cells — no cartilage.

d The right lung has three lobes, the left lung has two.

e Rt. atrium — tricuspid valve — rt. ventricle — pulmonary valve — pulmonary artery — pulmonary capillaries — pulmonary veins — left atrium — mitral valve — left ventricle.

f Bronchial arteries.

g Outer parietal pleura, inner visceral pleura.

h Oxygen present in the inspired air in the alveoli diffuses into the pulmonary capillaries, the pressure of oxygen in the alveoli being greater than that in the pulmonary capillaries. The pressure of carbon dioxide in the pulmonary capillaries is greater than that in the alveoli, so diffuses the other way i.e. from the capillaries to the alveoli.

i Minute air spaces forming the terminal end of the respiratory airways and through which the interchanges of gases can take place.

j This would prevent a pneumothorax, should the drainage tubes become disconnected.

k The bottle should never be lifted higher than bed-level, and it should be placed where it will not be accidently knocked over, at the same time it should not be pulling on the drainage tubes.

l To allow drainage of air and fluid from the chest on expiration.
The seal prevents air being sucked into the chest on inspiration, thus allowing restoration of the negative pleural pressure.

2.

a The potential space between the two layers of pleura, in health contains a thin film of serous fluid.

b A double layer of tissue (such as the pleura and peritoneum and pericardium). The presence of serous fluid between the layers prevents friction on movement.

c The layers of pleura are in close contact with each other in health, the space between is termed the potential space, it is possible for air or fluid to accumulate between the layers thus separating them.

d The presence of air in the pleural cavity which causes the underlying lung to collapse.

e Displacement of the mediastinum caused by a build-up of pressure on one side of the chest — as might occur with a 'tension' pneumothorax.

f Term to describe a terminal bronchiole and its divisions into the alveoli.

g The amount of exercise the patient can cope with before he shows signs of difficulty.

h The chief accessory muscles are the sterno-mastoid, scalene muscles and upper part of trapezius i.e. muscles of the shoulder girdle — used to raise the thoracic cage and increase the volume of the thorax. The pectorals are also used if the shoulder girdle is fixed.

i The alveolar ventilation must be distributed in such a way that it matches the pulmonary blood flow to all parts of the lung. If so each part of the lung has the correct ventilation/perfusion ratio.

j Placing the patient in the positions most suitable for drainage of pulmonary secretions from affected areas of lung by gravity.

k Unequal movements of the chest which occur when the two lungs are not working in unison as may occur in pneumothorax.

l The volume of each expiration × the number of breaths in one minute.

m A form of closed chest drainage, the draining tube attached to a glass tube, the end of which is submerged in water to form a seal.

n Difficulty in breathing experienced by the patient.

o The transudation of fluid into the pleural cavity e.g. as might occur from lung disease.

3.

a False	**e** False	**h** False
b False	**f** False	**i** False
c True	**g** True	**j** False
d False		

9 THE THYROID GLAND

The objectives for this section are to state:
1 The regional and applied A & P of the thyroid gland.
2 The investigations, management and care of patients, undergoing surgery of this gland.

The thyroid gland lies in the lower part of the neck between the two sterno-mastoid muscles. It consists of two lobes lying either side of the trachea and oesophagus and is joined in front of the trachea by a narrow band of tissue called the isthmus.

The gland consists of a number of closed vesicles which contain a colloidal substance called thyroglobin in which is stored thyroid hormone. The thyroid gland is richly supplied by blood from branches of the carotid and sub-clavian arteries. The muscles controlling the vocal cords are supplied by the recurrent laryngeal nerve which passes up behind the thyroid gland. Under the control of the thyroid stimulating hormone from the anterior pituitary gland the thyroid gland produces and releases into the blood three hormones:—

a	**Thyroxine**	essential for normal growth in infancy
b	**Tri-iodothyronine**	and normal metabolism in adulthood.
c	**Calcitonin**	lowers serum calcium by promoting excretion in urine and movement into bone.

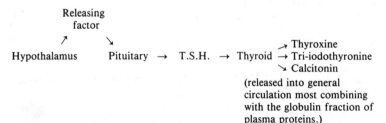

Normal activity of thyroid gland depends on the presence of iodine in the diet which it absorbs from the blood.

The parathyroid glands of which there are four, lie behind the thyroid gland. They secrete a substance called **parathormone** which maintains normal levels of calcium in the blood.

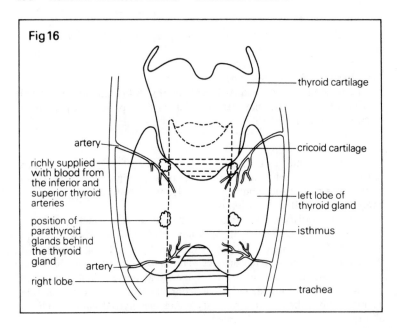

Fig 16

- thyroid cartilage
- cricoid cartilage
- left lobe of thyroid gland
- isthmus
- trachea

artery

richly supplied with blood from the inferior and superior thyroid arteries

position of parathyroid glands behind the thyroid gland

artery

right lobe

Goitre

This is swelling of the gland and may be **toxic** or **non toxic** and may be due to:

a lack of iodine in the diet

b over-activity of the secretory vesicles.

Surgery is indicated if the patient complains of:

1 Pressure symptoms

    a Dysphagia — difficulty in swallowing caused by pressure of the enlarged gland on the oesophagus.

    b Dyspnoea — difficulty in breathing caused by pressure of the enlarged gland on the trachea which may be displaced.

    c Voice change — hoarseness of voice caused by pressure on recurrent laryngeal nerve.

2 Symptoms which give rise to suspicion of malignancy.

3 Cosmetic reasons

4 Development of toxic changes (thyrotoxicosis).

Thyrotoxicosis

This is the excessive secretion of the thyroid hormone **thyroxine**. (the gland may or may not be enlarged).

Effect of excess thyroxine in the circulation:

Acceleration of metabolic rate:

Increased heat production — excessive sweating — hands warm and moist — patient prefers cold to hot weather.

Increased appetite even though there may be weight loss — patient may complain of tiring quickly.

Restlessness, nervousness, irritability — patient may get agitated or excited very quickly.

Tremors of fingers as seen when hands are outstretched.

Increased gastro-intestinal activity resulting in diarrhoea and vomiting.

Menstrual disturbances.

Eye changes — exophthalmus — the eyes are staring and protruding (thought to be due to a substance released by the anterior pituitary).

Cardio-vascular system

Heart and pulse rate increase, patient may complain of palpitations and shortness of breath on exertion — later irregularity of heart rhythm (atrial fibrillation) may lead on to cardiac failure.

Diastolic blood pressure is lowered due to widespread vasodilation.

Nursing care of patient undergoing thyroidectomy for thyrotoxicosis

Pre-operative

Drugs

The patient will probably have been admitted as a booked admission 2–10 days before intended date for operation, having received a course of antithyroid drugs (e.g. **carbimazole**) as an outpatient. These drugs will have been taken for several weeks and may or may not be continued up until the day of operation. **Lugol's iodine** is given in milk three times a day for up to 10 days prior to operation day, this reduces the vascularity of the gland.

The patient should have been rendered **euthyroid (normal thyroid activity)** before the operation, however there might still be tension and the patient may need sedation (e.g. **valium**) in order to rest. Ascertaining the particular aspects of the hospitalization which are worrying the patient, explanation of procedures and expected sequence of events will do much to help the patient relax.

The patient may have disturbances of cardiac rate and rhythm as a result of excessive thyroid activity for which a beta blocker (e.g. **propanolol** and/or **digoxin**) may have been prescribed.

Observations

a Daily temperature, respiration and blood pressure unless otherwise indicated.

b 2–4 hourly pulse rate including **sleeping pulse**

c Heart rate (apex beat) may be necessary.

d Urine Test — glycosuria may be present due to disturbed sugar metabolism.

e Eyes — soreness of eyes due to corneal ulceration caused by exophthalmos may require instillation of drops.

Specific investigations

Chest X-ray and **neck X-ray** (to determine position of trachea)

Electrocardiograph

Indirect laryngoscopy to establish degree of mobility of vocal cords

Routine blood examination + thyroid function tests — serum protein, iodine is high in thyrotoxicosis, + serum cholesterol — may be low.

Specific preparation

The neck, upper part of chest and axilla need to be shaved.

Operation

Sub-total thyroidectomy — up to 90% of the gland may be removed, care being taken not to injure the recurrent laryngeal nerves or the parathyroid glands. The wound is closed and drained through a tube (commonly a vacuum drainage apparatus).

Post-operative

Once the patient has fully recovered from the anaesthetic and vital signs are satisfactory, she is sat up with head and neck well-supported by pillows.

Intravenous infusion is usually continued until the patient is taking adequate oral fluids — small amounts of cool fluids can be encouraged as soon as possible and increased appropriately.

Specific observations

Initially these should be recorded at 1 hourly intervals (at least).

1 Temperature

2 Pulse (particular note of rate and rhythym)

a rise in temperature, sweating, tremor, and a rapid irregular pulse may be indicative of thyroid crisis.

3 Respirations — rate, and particularly alterations in character:

Signs of difficulty in breathing may indicate pressure on the trachea and be haematoma.

4 Blood pressure.
5 Wound — observe:
   a dressing for signs of bleeding,
   b area around wound for swelling or bruising. If present, check drainage tube is patent, gently mark area of discoloration on skin, inform person in charge at once (wound may need to be re-opened),
   c note that blood is not being lost and trickling down back of neck.

Frequency of recordings will then be altered according to patient's general condition.

Patients often complain of headache following thyroidectomy.

a Suitable analgesia will need to be prescribed.
b Sedation for 24 hours is usually prescribed.
c Hoarseness of voice is often distressing for the patient. It is important to reassure her that this will improve. Moist inhalations have a soothing effect.
d Soreness of the throat is helped by plenty of cool oral fluids, Asprin gargles can be prescribed if necessary.

The patient should be encouraged to mobilize the day following operation. Serum calcium levels will be estimated post-operatively, the patient must be observed for signs of **tetany** (tingling, numbness of face and hands and twitching of muscles). The doctor may elicit Trouseau's sign and Chvostek's sign. Low post-operative calcium is treated by i.v. calcium gluconate or oral calcium lactate.

The drainage tube is removed at approximately 48 hours.

If clips have been used for wound closure, alternate clips are removed on the 3rd day and the remainder on the 4th day. If sutures were used, they are removed on the 4th or 5th day.

Check indirect laryngoscopy is performed prior to discharge home.

An out-patient appointment is arranged for 4–6 weeks.

Practice Questions

Test 9

1. **Answer the following questions:**
   a How many lobes has the thyroid gland?
   b Where is the gland situated?
   c What is the isthmus?
   d Which arteries directly supply the thyroid gland?
   e The thyroid is drained by which veins?
   f The muscles controlling the vocal cords are supplied by which nerve?
   g Where are the parathyroid glands in relation to the thyroid?
   h Name the three thyroid hormones?
   i Name the parathyroid hormone.
   j What is an enlargement of the thyroid known as?
   k What may a thyroid enlargement be due to?
   l What is latent tetany and how may it be determined?
   m Why is a neck X-ray performed pre-operatively?
   n Briefly, how may an overactive thyroid lead to cardiac failure?
   o Why is potassium iodide (Lugol's iodine) given pre-operatively?
   p Why is an indirect laryngoscopy performed before and following thyroidectomy?

2. **What do you understand by the following terms?**
   a Thyrotoxicosis (Graves Disease)
   b Myxoedema
   c Exophthalmos
   d Dysphagia
   e Thyroid crisis
   f Tetany
   g Antithyroid drug (Carbimazole)
   h Sleeping Pulse
   i Pulse deficit
   j Basal metabolic rate
   k Euthyroid
   l Endemic goitre
   m Colloid
   n Thyroxine
   o Calcitonin
   p Laryngeal stridor

3. Mark the following statements true or false.

   a Thyroid stimulating hormone is released by the hypothalamus.

   b The patient with tracheal compression may complain of dysphagia.

   c Exophthalmos is caused by excess circulating thyroxine.

   d The hypothalamus secretes a releasing factor which stimulates the pituitary gland.

   e Thyroid stimulating hormone is secreted by the post pituitary gland.

   f Recurrent laryngeal nerve injury may result in permanent voice loss and tracheostomy.

   g A positive Chvostek's sign is indicative of hypothyroidism.

   h Calcitonin is a hormone secreted by the parathyroid gland.

   i Parathormone maintains normal levels of blood calcium.

   j The thyroid gland lies behind the trachea and in front of the oesophagus.

   k Thyroxine lowers the blood cholesterol level by increasing the excretion of cholesterol in the bile.

   l Oral fluids should be withheld until swallowing is no longer painful, post-operatively.

  m Low temperature, rapid thready pulse and restlessness following thyroidectomy is indicative of thyroid crisis.

   n Tetany may be a long term complication of total thyroidectomy.

   o Myxoedema may be a long term complication of total thyroidectomy.

   p Iodine should be omitted from the diet following thyroidectomy.

Answers to Test 9

1. a Two

   b In the lower part of the neck between the two sternomastoid muscles.

   c The band of tissue lying in front of the trachea that connects the two thyroid lobes.

   d Inferior and superior thyroid arteries.

   e Thyroid veins into the internal jugular vein.

   f Recurrent laryngeal nerve.

   g They lie behind the thyroid gland and are situated one to each pole.

   h Thyroxine, Tri-iodothyronine, Calcitonin.

   i Parathormone.

   j Goitre.

   k Lack of iodine uptake from diet — non-toxic goitre, excess secretion of thyroid hormones — toxic goitre tumour.

l Lowered serum calcium which has yet to manifest itself clinically.

m To establish the position of the trachea — it may be displaced by an enlarged thyroid gland.

n Acceleration of metabolic activity requires an increased oxygen uptake — the heart and pulse rate increases to meet the demand. This together with the effect of the thyroid hormones on the sympathetic nervous sytem may lead to arrythmias such as atrial fibrillation or ectopic beats.

o To reduce the vascularity of the gland.

p To establish whether there is normal movement of the vocal cords.

2. a Symptoms of increased metabolic activity that arise as a result of an excess secretion of thyroxine by the thyroid gland.

b Symptoms of decreased metabolic activity that arise as a result of under-secretion of the thyroid gland.

c Protrusion of the eyeball, sometimes seen in thyrotoxicosis — thought to be due to a substance released by the anterior pituitory gland.

d Difficulty in swallowing which might be a pressure symptom — an enlarged thyroid gland pressing on the oesophagus.

e A state of great agitation with extreme tachycardia and hyperpyrexia due to a sudden rise in metabolic rate — thought to be caused by a sudden surge of thyroxine into the bloodstream during operation.

f Increased excitability of the nerves and neuro-muscular functions causing muscular twitching and spasm — due to a fall in the plasma calcium level.

g Carbimazole belongs to the thiouracil group of drugs which act by inhibiting the formation of thyroxine in the thyroid gland in order to control the symptoms of thyrotoxicosis.

h Observation of the sleeping pulse is requested prior to thyroidectomy. It would remain raised if the patient's metabolic rate was still high.

i The difference between the pulse rate and apex beat — seen in atrial fibrillation — this might occur in thyrotoxicosis.

j This is the calorie requirement of the body when there is a state of complete mental and physical rest 12–18 hours after a meal so that digestion and absorption have been completed. Estimated by measuring the O_2 intake and CO_2 output in breathing.

k A condition in which the thyroid gland is functioning normally.

l Seen in some inland areas of the world (Switzerland, Himalayas) where there is lack of iodine in the water and soil.

m A gelatinous substance — in this instance found in the vesicles of the thyroid gland and in which thyroglobulin is stored.

n The iodine-containing hormone secreted by the thyroid gland. It is essential for normal growth in infancy and normal metabolism in adulthood.

o This hormone is secreted by the thyroid gland and its action is to lower the blood calcium by trapping the calcium in bone.

p A high-pitched harsh sound in breathing caused by air passing through constricted air passages — in this instance caused by constriction within the larynx.

3. a False   **g** True   **l** False
  b False   **h** False   **m** False
  c False   **i** True   **n** False
  d True   **j** False   **o** True
  e False   **k** True   **p** False
  f True

10 THE BREASTS

The objectives of this section are to state:
1 The applied and regional A & P of the breast.
2 Conditions common in the breast.
3 Investigation, management and care of patients undergoing breast surgery.

The breasts are undeveloped in both sexes until puberty. At this time the female breasts develop in response to an increase in circulating anterior pituitary and ovarian hormones.

The breasts are situated in the superficial fascia of the anterior chest wall and lie mainly over the pectoralis major muscle. Each extends from above the 2nd to the 6th rib and from the lateral border of the sternum to the mid-axillary line. The upper outer quadrant of each breast extends up into the axilla like a tail. Supporting ligaments extend from the skin through the breast tissue to the fascia.

The mature female breast is composed of 15–20 lobes arranged radially around the nipple. Each lobe consists of an arrangement of secreting cells and a system of ducts. A duct from each lobe opens onto the nipple. The pigmented area around the nipple is called the areola.

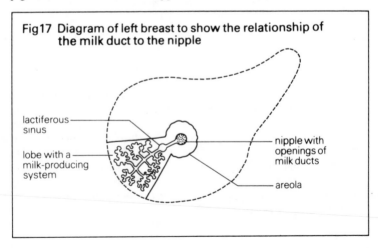

Fig17 Diagram of left breast to show the relationship of the milk duct to the nipple

lactiferous sinus

lobe with a milk-producing system

nipple with openings of milk ducts

areola

The breasts are richly supplied with blood from the **internal and external mammary** arteries and from branches of the **intercostal** arteries. Venous drainage is via a network of veins which drain into the **internal mammary** and **axillary veins**.

The lymphatic vessels of the breast drain lymph **medially to the anterior mediastinal** glands, **laterally to the axillary** glands and to glands in **the liver**. The lymphatics of the two breasts communicate with each other.

Cancer spreads early via these lymphatic vessels, thus, establishing whether there is lymph node involvement of these vessels is important when planning treatment of breast disease.

The nipple

The nipple is an erectile structure and **retraction of the nipple is** of diagnostic importance.

1   As a developmental abnormality — retraction may occur at puberty. It may be bilateral and may be remedied by regular daily manipulation and drawing out of the nipple. If not remedied, the condition may limit effective breast feeding and may predispose to infection and abscess formation.

2   Recent retraction occurring in adult woman is unfortunately frequently associated with scirrhous carcinoma of the breast.

It is therefore important to establish how long the nipple has been retracted.

Discharge from the nipple

This is another common symptom of breast disease. Discharge may be bloodstained, serous, purulent, yellowish brown or green, or milky.

The breasts are subject to menstrual cyclical changes associated with fluctuations in the circulating hormone levels. Enlargement and retrogression should occur evenly throughout the breast tissue. Occasionally, however, an imbalance of this process occurs, with a resulting irregularity or lumpiness of the breast tissue. This condition is known as **fibroadenosis**. If the patient presents with diffuse lumpiness of the breast tissue, she would not be submitted for surgery but kept under supervision, taught self examination of the breast and advised to report to her doctor if she feels any localised lump. If a localised lump can be palpated, it would be excised and sent for histological examination. Cysts may require aspirating.

The three most common symptoms of breast disease are:

1   A lump in the breast
2   A discharge or bleeding from the nipple
3   Pain

The patient may also present with a swelling in the axilla, nipple retraction, alterations in the shape or outline of the breast or inflammation of the breast.

Diagnosis is made following careful **physical medical examination, radiological** and **laboratory examination**.

Inspection and palpation of the breast is essential.

Mammography and Thermography may be indicated.

Tissue or discharge specimens may be sent for histological examination. Acute inflammatory disease of the breast may be treated with antibiotics, therapy, or if a localised abscess is present, by drainage. Benign breast tumours, (fibroadenomas and intraduct papilloma) are treated by excision and histological confirmation of the diagnosis.

The treatment of malignant breast tumours depends on the **staging** (or degree of spread) of the disease.

STAGE 1: Tumour confined to the breast

STAGE 2: Tumour in the breast and enlarged mobile axillary nodes

STAGE 3: Tumour and/or nodes are fixed superficially or deeply

STAGE 4: Distant metastasis are present.

A knowledge of how breast cancer may spread will help the nurses understand the stages above.

1   **Direct invasion** of surrounding tissues — this may result in puckering of the skin, nipple retraction or even ulceration superficially. Deep invasion may involve the underlying muscle and chest wall.

2   **Lymphatic spread** — superficially leads to the appearance of 'peau d'orange'. Along the lymph vessels to the internal mammary and axillary nodes. Later spread involves the supraclavicular and more distant lymph nodes.

3   Blood spread to the lungs, liver and bones.

4   Across cavities — pleural and peritoneal seeding.

Care of the patient with a breast lump
Pre-operation

The patient admitted to hospital with a breast lump is usually worried that the lump will prove to be malignant. This anxiety is not confined to the patient alone, but often to her near relatives. All must be done to help the patient cope with the situation during the investigative period but it is difficult and frequently impossible to allay the patient's fears completely. Following routine examination and palpation of the breast, the situation should be discussed fully with the patient.

a It may simply be at this stage that no further investigations are needed other than an excision biopsy under anaesthesia. A consent form is signed accordingly and the patient prepared for surgery usually for the following day. After a simple excision biopsy procedure, the patient is usually allowed home within two days and returns to the hospital for removal of sutures/clips and the biopsy result.

b If there is a suspicion that the lump is malignant, further investigations may be carried out prior to surgical intervention.

Blood examination (a low Hb may be suggestive of widespread bone involvement).

Chest X-ray

Mammography and/or **Thermography** — these may show a tumour that could not be palpated.

Skeletal survey — may yield distant bony metastases.

A decision can then be made on the course of treatment, and whether it aims to be curative or palliative.

Stages 1 and 2

Operative treatment ranges between the following:

Removal of the lump only

Removal of the lump and axillary node biopsy

Segmental mastectomy and axillary node biopsy

Simple mastectomy and axillary node biopsy

Simple mastectomy with axillary node clearance

Radical mastectomy

These procedures may be preceded or followed by radiotherapy, and sometimes radiotherapy to, or removal of, the ovaries is considered.

Mastectomy — pre-operation

Much reassurance will be needed during the days preceding operation. Every opportunity must be afforded the patient to allow her to discuss her anxieties. It is often wise to involve her close relatives in these pre-operative discussions so that all are in a more effective position to give appropriate support to one another. The patient should be assured of the excellent cosmetic results gained from skilled prosthesis fittings. Arrangements can be made for her to meet the person dealing with breast prosthesis before operation so that personal details and fears can be discussed and measurements taken. Some hospitals arrange for the patient to be visited by a person who has already undergone mastectomy, this often proves to be a great psychological boost to the patient.

A full explanation of what to expect after the operation is given and the physiotherapist teaches the patient the specific exercises she will expect her to perform.

The consent form for operation may be one of the following.

a   For excision of breast lump, then return to ward and consent for further surgery if necessary.

b   For excision of breast lump, urgent histological examination of tissue whilst patient is still under anaesthesia and immediate follow-on to mastectomy if necessary.

c   For full procedure, that is simple mastectomy or radical mastectomy.

The skin of the appropriate side is marked by the doctor.

Both axillae are shaved prior to general preparation.

Post-operation

The patient returns to the ward with an intravenous infusion or transfusion *in situ*. I.v. replacement is usually discontinued after 12–24 hours when the patient's condition is satisfactory. There is usually no restriction on oral intake.

There may be a pressure dressing over the breast wound, this may be removed after 24–48 hours. The wound is usually drained by two drainage tubes, one placed medially and the other laterally in the axilla. It is important that maximum drainage is promoted since an accumulation of fluid under the wound can predispose to wound breakdown and necrosis (this is because the wound is often closed under tension), and in the axillary pocket to infection. The drainage tubes are not removed until drainage ceases, the medial usually draining less than the lateral.

The patient is supported in the sitting position as soon as her condition allows, the arm on the affected side positioned comfortably and elevated slightly on a pillow.

Adequate analgesia and/or sedation should be ensured, the patient often becoming 'weepy' when full realization of the operation occurs.

The patient is assisted out of bed after 24 hours and ambulation and self-care encouraged appropriately to the patient's response. The physiotherapist and nursing staff encourage **gentle** hand, arm and shoulder exercises on the first day, increasing the range and movement gradually throughout the post-operative period in accordance with the wishes of the surgeon. The patient usually feels less anxious about doing these exercises when drainage tubes have been removed (usually 3–6th day).

Sutures are removed 7–10th day.

Wound dressing times are usually traumatic for the patient because she has to come to terms with her altered body image. The help that the nurse gives to enable the patient to cope, will vary with each patient's response. It is for this reason that many centres arrange early fitting and wearing of breast prosthesis before the patient is ready for discharge home.

Post-operative radiotherapy will depend on the histology findings and whether it is considered that all malignant tissue has been excised. Again, the patient needs much support since she often feels her need for this type of follow-up treatment as being an ominous sign. Surgical follow-up appointments will be continued.

Stage 3

At this stage the disease has spread beyond the breast and although surgery to the breast is sometimes considered, palliative local radiotherapy is usually the treatment of choice.

Stage 4 — and recurrences after previous mastectomy

A number of measures may be employed.

Local radiotherapy to recurrent deposits in scar or solitary deposits elsewhere.

If the disease is widespread, **hormone therapy** or **hormone surgery** is considered. This is based on the fact that about 30% of all breast tumours are hormone dependant. Removal of or interference with the actions of these hormones can sometimes lead to a regression of tumour growth giving temporary palliative relief.

Cytotoxic therapy.

Practice Questions
Test 10

1. Answer the following questions.
1. Name the three main types of tissue that comprise the mammary glands.
2. How many lobes has a normal mature breast?
3. Where are the milk-producing alveoli situated?
4. What is the purpose of the lactiferous sinus?
5. The breasts lie mainly over which muscle?
6. Describe the contours (extent of breast tissue) of the breast.
7. Where is the areola?
8. Name the glands in the areola.
9. What type are the above glands?
10. Name the hormone(s) that affect breast development at puberty.
11. Describe the lymphatic drainage of the breast.
12. What are said to be the 3 most common symptoms of breast disease?
13. Why is nipple retraction of important diagnostic significance?
14. Describe the blood supply to the breast.
15. Briefly outline the 4 stages of malignant breast cancer.
16. Briefly outline the ways in which malignant breast disease can spread.

2. What do you understand by the following terms?
1. Simple mastectomy.
2. Radical mastectomy.
3. Axillary node clearance.
4. P'eau d'orange.
5. Fibroadenosis.
6. Mammography.
7. Thermogram.
8. Skeletal Survey.
9. T.N.M. Classification.
10. Lymphoedema.

1. *Answers to Test 10*
1. Glandular, fibrous fatty
2. 15–20
3. Deep within the breast, each of the breast lobes is divided into many lobules which consist of milk excreting units known as alveoli.
4. The main milk duct has a dilation just below the surface called the lactiferous sinus. Milk collected in this sinus is available for the baby by sucking.

5. Pectoralis major.
6. From 2nd to 6th rib and from lateral border of sternum to the mid-axillary line, the upper outer quadrant extending up towards the axilla.
7. The areola is the pigmented area around the nipple.
8. Montgomery's tubules.
9. They are sebaceous glands which lubricate the nipple in pregnancy.
10. At puberty the breasts develop in response to stimulation of oestrogens.
11. Lymph is drained mainly medially to the anterior mediastinal glands, and laterally to the axillary glands.
12. A lump in the breast, a discharge or bleeding from the nipple and pain.
13. Recent nipple retraction in the adult woman might be indicative of breast malignancy.
14. Supplied by the internal and external mammary arteries and the upper intercostal arteries.
15. Stage 1. Tumour confined to the breast.
     2. Tumour in the breast plus enlarged mobile axillary nodes.
     3. Tumour and/or nodes fixed.
     4. Presence of distant metastases.
16. Via the bloodstream.
    Via the lymphatic stream.
    By direct invasion.
    Across cavities.

2.
1. Removal of the breast tissue alone, leaving the lymphatics and pectoral muscles intact.
2. Removal of the complete breast, underlying pectoral muscles, axillary lymphatics and lymph nodes.
3. Removal of the axillary nodes usually combined with mastectomy.
4. Superficial lymphatic blockage causing dimpling and 'orange peel' appearance of the breast skin.
5. Diffuse lumpiness of breast tissue that may result from the cyclical changes that occur in breast tissue.
6. A specific radiographic procedure which shows areas of increased density in breast tissue.
7. A method of estimating changes in skin temperature with an infra-red camera. The skin overlying tumours is warmer than over normal areas.

8. A series of X-rays of various parts of the skeleton to elecite distant bony metastases.

9. A method of classifying the stages of breast cancer
   T — Tumour
   N — Node
   M — Metastases

10. A late complication of radical mastectomy — gross swelling of the arm on the side of mastectomy as a result of removal of the axillary lymphatics.

11 BLOOD VESSELS

The objectives of this section are to state:
1 The regional and applied structure and function of blood vessels.
2 The diseases most commonly associated with blood vessels and the ways in which they interfere with normal function.
3 The management of the individual undergoing investigation and treatment of conditions of the blood vessels.

Fig. 18 (a, b, c, d) is a diagrammatic representation of the structure of arteries, veins and capillaries. Revise with textbooks and your lecture notes. Learn to draw line diagrams and label them correctly.

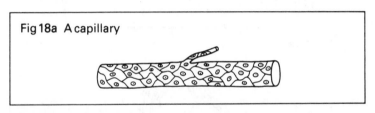

Fig 18a A capillary

The wall of a capillary is composed of a single layer of endothelial cells permeable to water and crystaloids, but only semi-permeable to plasma proteins. The lumen of the capillary just allows red blood cells to pass. The function of the capillaries, by a process of osmosis and diffusion, is to convey oxygen and nutrition to the tissue cells and carry carbon dioxide and waste products of cell metabolism away from the cells. The osmotic pressure of plasma proteins and tissue fluids and the hydrostatic pressure of blood in the capillaries regulate this function. Oedema or swelling occurs when there is an imbalance in these two factors.

There are several types of blood vessels:
Arteries and arterioles carry blood oxygen and nutrition away from the heart to the tissues via the capillaries. Veinules and veins carry blood, carbon dioxide and waste products (via the capillaries) away from the tissues to the heart. Arteries and veins have a similar basic structure:
a Tunica Intima — an inner layer of flat squamous cells.
b Tunica Media — a middle layer of elastic and muscle tissue.
c Tunica Adventitia — an outer fibrous protective layer.

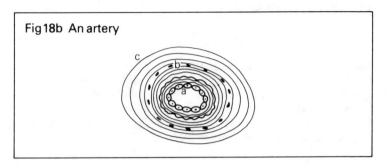

Fig 18b An artery

Key **Artery**
A — Tunica Intima
B — Tunica Media
C — Tunica Adventitia

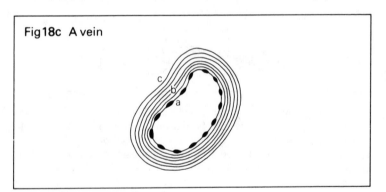

Fig 18c A vein

Key **Vein**
A — Tunica Intima
B — Tunica Media
C — Tunica Adventitia

The vessels are adapted to fulfil their functions:

a Veins have a thin weak middle layer which will collapse if cut. Most veins have valves which prevent the backflow of blood. Incompetent veins give rise to varicose veins.

b Arteries have a strong middle layer and remain open if cut. Large arteries have more elastic tissues i.e. the aorta has to accommodate

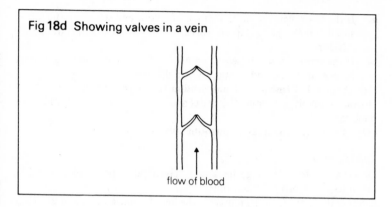

Fig 18d Showing valves in a vein

flow of blood

blood from the heart. Arterioles have more muscle, they are responsible for the peripheral resistance of blood pressure.

Disease of arteries

Emboli

An embolism is a foreign body which circulates in the blood stream lodging in a small vessel, eventually obstruction to blood flow results. Blockage of end arteries can cause dramatic effects i.e. in the retina, blindness, in the small intestine, gangrene of gut, in the brain, stroke. Emboli may be:

a simple due to blood clots, fat, air or vegetation from cardiac valves in rheumatic heart disease.

b Infective due to infected blood clot or masses of bacteria.

c Malignant due to masses of carcinomatous cells.

Common causes of emboli are from atrial fibrillation, in rheumatic heart disease vegetation dislodges from heart valves, in myocardial infarction blood clots dislodge from the ventricles.

A typical history of arterial blockage in a limb is sudden pain. The limb becomes white, cold and pulseless, sensation may disappear and the muscles become paralysed.

On admission the patient is made as comfortable as possible (the pain is severe). Expose the limb to room temperature, take the vital signs and observe the limb for impairment of circulation. As soon as the diagnosis is made heparin will be given to prevent further extension of the clot. The limb must be observed and observations charted.

F

a   If the limb seems to have a return of colour and sensation the blood supply may be adequate because of a collateral circulation developing.

b   If the limb is cold, pulseless, painful and paralysed these signs must be urgently reported as surgery is indicated.

(See chapter 1. Principles of preparation for surgery.)

Operation involves opening the vessel and inserting a Fogarty Catheter to remove the clot.

(See chapter 1. Principles of post-operative care.)

Specific care

Observation for bleeding, heparin is given post-operatively, blood is taken to check prothrombin time.

Observe the limb. Colour, pulses. If the limb becomes white and pulseless the doctor must be informed immediately.

After successful embolectomy the cause of the embolus is treated if possible.

Trauma to arteries

Arteries may be injured by closed or open trauma

Closed injuries include pressure from too tightly applied plaster of paris, a tourniquet left on too long or a bone splinter in closed fracture.

Signs and symptoms are: Pain, pallor, pulselessness, paraesthesia and paralysis. Observations must be made frequently of newly applied plaster of paris. Plaster charts should be kept, any sign of a too tight plaster should be reported. Raising the limb may reduce swelling or the plaster may need to be bi-valved. If a tourniquet is applied it should be released at regular intervals and records kept of the state of the limb, deterioration in the limb must be reported. Fractures should be reduced under general anaesthetic.

Open injuries

Arteries may be injured by compound fractures, gunshot wounds or stabbing. Treatment is of the cause.

Varicose veins

It is said that varicose veins are due to the fact that man has assumed an upright position in evolution.

Varicose veins may occur

1   In the anal canal — haemorrhoids

2   In the oesophagus — varices

3   In the testes — varicocele
4   Most commonly in the legs
a   Primary varicose veins — the biggest group of people, mostly female, suffer from valve defect.
b   Secondary varicose veins
   i   due to deep vein thrombosis
   ii   due to raised venous pressure as in pregnancy or pelvic tumour.

Signs and symptoms: Unsightly and prominent veins, pain or swelling of the legs. Ulcers may form around the ankles.

Complications 1. Haemorrhage, 2. Phlebitis, 3. Ulceration.

Treatment
1   Injection of sclerosing agent, compression bandages are applied. The patient is encouraged to exercise and lose weight if necessary.
2   Elastic supportive stockings may be prescribed for the elderly or unfit.
3   Surgical intervention:
   a   Stripping
   b   Ligation of veins

(See chapter 1 for basic principles of pre and post-operative care.)

Specific care
1   Raise the foot end of the bed to help reduce swelling.
2   Inspect the feet for swelling and temperature.
3   Make sure the bandages are not obstructing blood flow.
4   Observe bandages for bleeding.

Before discharge the patient is fitted with elastic stockings and instructed how to apply them.

Ulceration

An ulcer is a local defect or excavation of an organ produced by shedding or sloughing of the surface tissues due to any cause. Most frequently seen in the skin or gastro-intestinal tract.

Ulcers may be classified as:
1   Non-specific pressure sores, dental ulcer,
2   Specific relating to peptic ulcers, syphilitic ulcers
3   Malignant ulcers, skin rodent ulcers.

Treatment of ulcers depend on the cause e.g. for varicose ulcers, pressure dressings are applied. Generally the patient is put to bed, the ulcer is kept clean and dry and a good diet is given.

Gangrene

Gangrene is death of a large area of tissue combined with putrefaction. Signs and symptoms are:

1 Pulselessness
2 Cold
3 Loss of sensation
4 Loss of function
5 Colour change depending on type of gangrene i.e. moist or dry gangrene.

Dry Gangrene occurs when blood supply is gradually diminished i.e. arteriosclerosis. The part becomes dry, wrinkled, discoloured from disintegration of haemoglobin and greasy to touch.

Moist Gangrene occurs when an artery is suddenly blocked e.g. by an embolus or when venous as well as arterial obstruction occurs. Infection and putrefaction usually follows. The affected part becomes swollen and discoloured. The epidermis may be raised in blobs.

Varieties of gangrene

1 Symptomatic:
   a Reynards disease
   b Ergot poisoning
   c Senile
   d Thrombosis
   e Embolism
   f Diabetes
2 Infective:
   Gas gangrene
   Carbuncles
   Boils
3 Traumatic:
   Strangulated bowel
   Pressure sores
4 Physical
   Burns
   Scalds
   Frost bite.

Nursing Care: to observe changes carefully:

a expose the limb, **b** cool with a fan, **c** elevate the limb to increase venous return and support the patient generally in this ordeal. Give analgesics when necessary.

Specific treatments of the cause.

i   Diabetes has to be controlled.

ii Embolism removed.

iii Gas gangrene is treated with large doses of antibiotics and hyperbaric oxygen.

iv Senile gangrene, care of the feet is important. If the blood supply is known to be good, amputation of the affected limb is performed eventually.

Practice Questions

Test 11

Test your comprehension of this section of the work. Answer the questions then check your answers.

1. What is the function of the capillaries?
2. Why do some arteries have a predominance of elastic tissue?
3. How do veins differ from arteries?
4. What is the function of arteries and veins?
5. What does emboli mean?
6. State the signs and symptoms of embolic obstruction in a limb.
7. State the possible causes of trauma to arteries.
8. What is the difference between dry and moist gangrene?
9. Where do varicose veins commonly occur? Name the sites.
10. State the treatment of varicose veins.
11. How are ulcers classified, give examples.
12. Define gangrene.
13. What are the varieties of gangrene, give examples.
14. Mrs Watkins aged 60 years falls in the ward and ruptures a varicose vein.
    a Describe the first aid treatment you would consider most appropriate to give to Mrs Watkins.
    b Describe how you would explain varicose veins to a junior nurse.
    c Describe the care Mrs Watkins would require after stripping and ligation of varicose veins.

Answers to Test 11

1. To convey O_2 water and nutrients to the tissues and to take CO_2 water and waste products away from the tissues by a process of osmosis and diffusion i.e. Osmotic pressure set up by plasma proteins remains constant in venous and arterial capillaries. 25 mm Hg. Blood pressure is higher in arterial capillaries about 40 mm Hg there is a pressure force of 15 mm Hg, blood pressure is lower in venous capillaries about 10 mm Hg therefore there is an effective suction of 25 mm Hg.
2. To fulfil the function large vessels receive and flush blood forward. Arterioles maintain peripheral resistance by controlling the flow of blood.
3. They have a thinner muscle coat, collapse when cut and many have valves.

4. To convey blood away from the heart to the tissues, to convey blood to the heart.

5. A foreign body circulating in the blood stream.

6. Sudden severe pain in the limb, which becomes pale, cold, loses sensation, may become pulseless and paralysed.

7. Closed injuries may result from closed fractures or too tight plaster of paris, or a tourniquet left on too long. Open injuries penetrating wounds, gunshot, stabbing.

8. Dry gangrene — a slow process resulting from a slowly diminishing blood supply as in arteriosclerosis or diabetes.
   Moist gangrene may occur from sudden obstruction by an emboli or when veins and arteries are obstructed.

9. In the legs, in the rectum and oesophagus.

10. Conservative. Reduction in weight loss. Injection with sclerosing agents. Support hose. Surgical stripping or ligation of veins.

11. **a** Non-specific — pressure sores **b** Specific — peptic ulcers.
    c Malignant — rodent ulcers

12. Death of tissue combined with putrefaction.

13. **a** Symptomatic i.e. thrombosis. **b** Infective — gas gangrene **c** Trauma — pressure sores, strangulated bowel **d** Physical — burns.

Model Answer to Question 14

a Reassure Mrs Watkins, send a helper to report the incident. Place Mrs Watkins in a comfortable recumbent position and raise her leg, apply pressure over the wound with a dressing. Keep the leg raised until the bleeding stops or abates. Apply a dressing over the wound and an elastic bandage. Bandage from the toes to above the wound keeping an even pressure. Take her vital signs and keep her at rest until she is seen by a doctor. The accident must be formally recorded.

b Varicose veins may be primary or secondary, and commonly due to valve defects. They may be secondary to deep vein thrombosis where the veins are patent but their valves are incompetent. The veins become distended and sometimes tortuous, the walls are thin and burst easily.

c Immediately post-operatively Mrs Watkins would be nursed in bed with the foot end of the bed elevated. The vital signs are taken and recorded. The feet are examined for swelling and pulses and colour are observed. The bandages should not be removed, if bleeding is observed a pressure dressing can be applied over the bandage. If the bandages are too tight they may be loosened. The raised foot end of bed should help relieve the swelling. Mrs Watkins should be encouraged to move in bed and as soon as possible to start walking placing the heel down first and deliberately stretching her toes. Firm elastic bandages will be applied and before Mrs Watkins is discharged home, clips and stitches will be removed and support hose supplied. She should be instructed to put on these very firm stockings first thing in the morning and to exercise her legs as much as she is able.

12 ADVICE FOR EXAMINATION PREPARATION

Start your preparation well in advance of the examination. Make a realistic plan of action that you will be able to achieve.

1. Decide how many hours each day you can set aside for study/revision 2 hours daily × 5 = 10 hours weekly.
2. Make a timetable and slot in all the subjects to be studied. The length of time you allocate depends on the level of difficulty.
3. Study in the same place each day. Sit at a desk or table and have the materials you need at hand i.e. paper, pencils, crayons, text books, lecture notes and a rubber. Write in pencil so that mistakes or unwanted notes can be erased (paper is expensive).
4. You must work at concentrating on your task, don't allow yourself to think of anything else so that you waste time.
5. If you are tired or upset, relax before attempting to settle.
6. Work at each of the goals you have set yourself as widely as you can.
7. Reward yourself when a goal is achieved so that you associate pleasure with studying.
8. Success is not a matter of luck but of good planning and self-discipline.
9. Learning is an active process so:
   a Study using a logical approach. Sequence the material and go from easy to more difficult concepts.
   b Don't try to learn chunks of material, skim the passage and try to understand. Underline key words or sentences. Use a dictionary.
   c Overlearn material and consciously recall and reinforce your memory. Commit your thoughts to paper.
   d Use mnemonics as a memory aid.
   e Ask yourself questions, apply the material, compare with management of actual patients you have nursed. Have discussions with friends/tutors.
   f Ask your tutors for help if you do not understand the relevance of a topic.
   g Learn to draw and label line drawings correctly.
   h Test yourself using past examination questions.
   i Get your relations or friends to ask you questions.

10. Cultivate a fast reading style. Use several textbooks with your notes. Make your own notes when you have analysed the meaning of a passage. Begin to read with a question in mind and ask yourself questions when you have read a paragraph/chapter. Read quickly then re-read.
11. What you want to achieve is efficiency of study with economy of effort.

Examination technique

1. Listen to the invigilator's instructions and follow them carefully. Have your number card signed and available for inspection. Be prepared with pens, pencils, a rubber and ruler.
2. Read the instructions on the front cover of the book and comply with them i.e. start a question on a fresh page, number your questions carefully, write legibly. Note how many questions are to be attempted, how much time is allowed etc.
3. Objective type questions test a wide area of knowledge, recognition and recall in a short time. Consider the questions carefully, and choose what you believe to be the correct answer from the distractors, do not just guess.
4. Essay questions test:
   a Knowledge
   b Comprehension
   c Application
   d Communication
   e Synthesis.
5. Read all the questions carefully on both sides of the paper, identify all parts of the question.
   a Don't be concerned that others have started to write.
   b Select the questions you feel most able to answer.
   c Tick your selection in order of sequence.
   d Analyse the setting of the question. Is the scene in hospital or the community? What is the importance of age, sex, marital/social status, environment, psychological well-being, needs of the patient in the examiner's mind.
   Underline these points and develop them.
   e Note the essential points that have to be made in your answer in the margin of the paper.
   f Pay attention to the weighting of each part of the question, these should help you plan the time to be spent on each part.

g Ten minutes spent in planning is the most effective way of using the examination time.

h When you start to write:

    i   answer the parts in order of a, b, c, d

    ii   write legibly, be logical (first things first)

    iii   concentrate on the main parts, don't waffle and repeat yourself

    iv   if a diagram is asked for make a clear line drawing and label it clearly

    v   leave time at the end for reading your answers.

Remember that a good essay has an introduction, a development and a conclusion, and should be clear and concise.

NOTES

NOTES

NOTES

NOTES

NOTES

NOTES

NOTES

NOTES

NOTES

NOTES

NOTES

NOTES

NOTES

NOTES

NOTES

NOTES

NOTES

NOTES

Exams?

Nurses don't have much time to study and revise. Which is why the study you can do has to count – has to be the *right* kind of study.

Celtic Revision Aids can help. With the new Celtic Revision Aids **Nursing Revision Notes** series, you can make the best of your training, by organising your study and revision properly, learning the *right* facts and the *right* way to apply them on the ward, and the *right* exam technique. The **Nursing Revision Notes** series is the *right* range for you, because the books are designed as a series of single subject practical nursing modules for use all the way through your course *and* in the vital revision period before your exams.

The **Nursing Revision Notes** series covers the most up-to-date syllabus requirements and will build rapidly into a complete set of titles for every subject you'll have to study during your nursing training.

Every title in the **Nursing Revision Notes** series is written by qualified and practising Nursing Tutors and Examiners — so you know that you're in the *right* hands!

Get it right!

Principles of Nursing   £1.95

This title takes the learner through, in detail, the nurse's responsibilities from the time of the patient's admission until discharge. The emphasis is on nursing care: nursing observations, the nurse's role in investigations, and ideas on how the nurse can help the patient overcome the various problems of hospitalization. Each chapter is finished by practice examination questions. The final chapter contains advice on examination preparation.

General Medical Nursing   £1.95

The introductory chapter defines the general principles of nursing care which apply for the nursing of all patients being treated for common medical conditions. Successive chapters deal with specific diseases and explain the disease process, the management of the disease, and the specific nursing care. At the end of each chapter are examination style questions, to test the learner's understanding of the material. The final chapter contains advice on examination preparation.

Surgical Nursing   £1.95

This book begins by defining the general principles of nursing care which apply in pre- and post- operative stages. The following chapters deal with different parts of the anatomy, explaining symptoms, investigations, surgery, and treatment that the patient with common problems needing surgical intervention will experience. Again, the emphasis is on nursing care in the surgical situation and, again, each chapter ends with a section of practice examination questions for nurse learners to test their understanding of the chapter. The final chapter contains advice on examination preparation.

Other books to be published in this series over the next two years are: Paediatric Nursing; Ear, Nose and Throat Nursing; Ophthalmic Nursing; Orthopaedic Nursing; Obstetric and Gynaecological Nursing; Psychiatric Nursing; Geriatric and Psychogeriatric Nursing.